Basic Surgical Techniques

An Illustrated Manual

Basic Surgical Techniques
An Illustrated Manual

A.K. Qayumi, M.D., Ph.D.

Professor of Surgery
University of British Columbia
Vancouver, BC, Canada

Emma J. Patterson, M.D., FRCSC

Assistant Editor
Laparoscopic Surgery Fellow
Mount Sinai Medical Center
New York, NY, USA

Q & Q Publishing 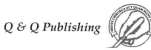 *Vancouver, Canada*

Basic Surgical Techniques: An Illustrated Manual

I would like to dedicate this book
to my mother, Rahima Dakik,
and my father, Dr. Khalik Qayumi

Preface

Mente Chirurga Act Quam Manu Armata
"The brain of a surgeon should act before his hand"

*B*asic surgical techniques and practical prospects of surgical skills have been traditionally learned through apprenticeship in medical schools. Today, due to an increasing number of students, residents, fellows, etc., the chance for medical students to learn basic surgical techniques through traditional apprenticeship has been reduced. The new problem-based learning curriculum in most North American medical schools looks for programs that consolidate and promote the practical aspects of medical knowledge. At the University of British Columbia Medical School a "Basic Surgical Technique" course has been developed that teaches medical students the fundamentals of surgical skills in a dry and wet laboratory environment before students start their surgical rotation. The "Basic Surgical Technique" program has made a significant improvement in the performance of medical students and interns. This improvement was evaluated by teachers, students themselves, and later confirmed by staff surgeons. This book is based on the "Basic Surgical Techniques" course and is written for the purpose of sharing the experience with the rest of the world.

Practical knowledge of surgical skills is scattered and, sometimes, hidden under a great deal of theory. The main objectives of this book are to describe and illustrate the practical aspect of surgical techniques in a consolidated, brief and practical format. Since this book is aimed at the delivery of practical knowledge, theoretical issues such as indication, contraindication, post-op care and other theoretical reasoning are not discussed.

The book consists of seven chapters aimed toward those who have just begun to learn surgery. The seven major areas covered are:

(1) Introduction to Basic Surgical Instruments
(2) Handling of Surgical Instruments
(3) Knot Tying Techniques
(4) Wound Management Techniques
(5) Aseptic Techniques and Operating Room Conduct
(6) Basic Surgical Procedures
(7) Laparoscopic Surgical Techniques

This book has over 500 coloured pictures illustrating the steps involved in surgical procedures. The chapters are organized to deliver knowledge in a stepwise progression 'from simple to more complicated' manner. This book may not be the wish list of all basic surgical techniques or procedures. Materials contained in this book are intended to be sufficient for the medical student to feel comfortable and confident in the surgical ward during his or her rotation as it pertains to practical aspects of surgical knowledge. This book is not only for those who have chosen surgery for their career, but rather, the content of this book is the absolute minimum practical knowledge required for any physician. The most unique feature of this book is the electronic format presented on an accompanied CD-ROM. This CD-ROM is by no means an electronic copy of the book, word for word and picture by picture - it is an interactive audiovisual aid to the book, and consists of more than 100 animated surgical procedures.

I gratefully acknowledge the help of my colleagues and staff of the Department of Surgery, my teachers and mentors, and especially Drs. A.D. Forward, G.F.O. Tyers, R.J. Finley and M.N. Mochnuk, as well as my students and everyone who participated in the completion of this book. In particular I would like to express my deepest appreciation to my wife Shahnaz, and my son Tarique, for being patient and helping me in the completion of this book.

A. K. Qayumi

Foreword

I was a medical student in the late 1950s. At that time, essentially no formal instruction was given to the student in basic surgical techniques. Instead, the student was expected to pick these techniques up during internship or in actual practice. Dr. Qayumi's Basic Surgical Techniques is the type of book that I wish had been available to me as a young student and surgical resident. I believe that basic surgical instruction is absolutely essential for all physicians, in particular young physicians who will face the "eternal challenge of how to do it right-the first time".

This book will find a favoured place in the library of each young student of medicine interested in an active surgical career.

A.D. Forward, MD, FRCSC
Associate Professor Emeritus
The University of British Columbia
Department of Surgery
Vancouver

With the introduction of new technologies at an ever-increasing rate, the practice of surgery is becoming steadily more complex. Members of the public as well as surgeons are quick to seek applications for these novel methods which, at first glance, seem to offer a potential surgical breakthrough. Usually, the potential major breakthrough is often expensive, adds to the complexity of the procedure and requires significant maintenance and storage. Ultimately, the new technology settles into a specific indication or a narrow application soon to be followed by yet another potential technical breakthrough.

Illustrated in this text, Dr. Qayumi outlines the essentials of basic surgical technique, all of which are necessary for any surgeon to carry out one's practice. The surgeon's workup, judgement and management can be undone by a single failure in surgical technique at any point in a long and complex procedure.

The trainee in surgery would do well to study and practice the techniques outlined in this text before presenting him or herself in the operating room. Not only would the trainee be allowed to perform some of these maneuvers under supervision in the clinical setting, but the student would likely get closer to the "action' in the operating room and thus see and do more thus enhancing the learning experience.

Included in this text are sections on sterile technique and, of increasing importance, safety techniques to prevent injury or contamination of the patient and operating room staff. This is now of critical importance as contraction of a communicable pathogen to the surgeon from the patient may alter the surgeon's career.

One technological breakthrough that is here to stay is minimal access surgery. These techniques which are finding increasing application in many subspecialties offer the patient less tissue trauma and scarring which translates into shorter rehabilitation times, less pain and expense with a better cosmetic result. Knowledge of basic laparoscopic techniques is essential even for the beginner trainee.

The slogan cut well, tie well, will do well *continues to be as important today as when modern surgical techniques were introduced over one hundred years ago. Today, new technologies offer no more than different ways of accomplishing the techniques outlined in this text.*

C.H. Scudamore, M.D. FRCSC
Associate Professor of Surgery
Head, Section of Hepatobiliary & Pancreatic Surgery
Surgical Director, Liver Transplant Program
Division of General Surgery, Department of Surgery

Student comments

"Basic Surgical Techniques *is an invaluable resource for any medical student. It will teach you everything you need to know to be comfortable and helpful in the operating room. It covers everything from how to tie surgical knots and hold surgical instruments to laparoscopic surgical techniques. This is a very easy to read text and the CD ROM which complements it makes this an interactive learning experience which can't be beat."*

Hamish Hwang

"Basic Surgical Techniques *is a concise review of basic surgical skills and knowledge required by medical students. Its vivid colour, simple illustrations bring the text to life. Reading this text will equip the medical student beginning their surgical clerkship to approach their first encounters in the operating room with greater confidence and skill, and thereby to enhance their learning experience. The CD is a unique educational aid in that it brings to life the dynamic nature of many of the techniques in a way that static textbook illustrations never could."*

Simon Pulfrev

"This text and CD would be an excellent primer for a MSI or Junior resident starting a surgical rotation. It covers basic techniques from knot tying to more complicated skills such as tracheostomy tube placement. The animations in the CD demonstrate each technique step by step so that they can be mastered rapidly. The text and CD would also be great resource as a refresher for the more complex techniques such as chest tube placement."

Jennifer Lush

"This manual is a good introduction for medical students starting their surgical clerkship. It would also be a good review source for non-surgical residents rotating through surgery. The accompanying CD-ROM provides a useful visual modality of learning that makes procedures that are difficult to visualize seem simple and straight-forward."

Zuheir Abrahams

"This manual would have been useful to have read before starting third year. It would have made the basic surgical skills workshops more time-efficient because less time would have been needed for explanation."

Clinton Chow

Contributors

Assistant Editor	Emma J. Patterson, M.D., FRCSC
Co-Authors	Alexander G. Nagy, M.D., FRCSC
	Judith S. Fialkow, R.N. BScN, CPN(C), (Chapter 5)
	Ctirad Kaděrábek, M.D.
Art Direction	Gary Cody
Artists	Dana Smith, Ryan Klak & Gary Cody
Technical Assistants	Joanne Dean, Melissa Chen & Tarique Qayumi
Audio Production	Anton Bernhardt
Narration	Cameron Bell
CD Production, Animation & Design	Ryan Klak
CD Assembly	Norm Elmore & Paul Planiden of RubberMind Media Ltd.

Contents

Chapter 1

Introduction to Basic Surgical Instruments

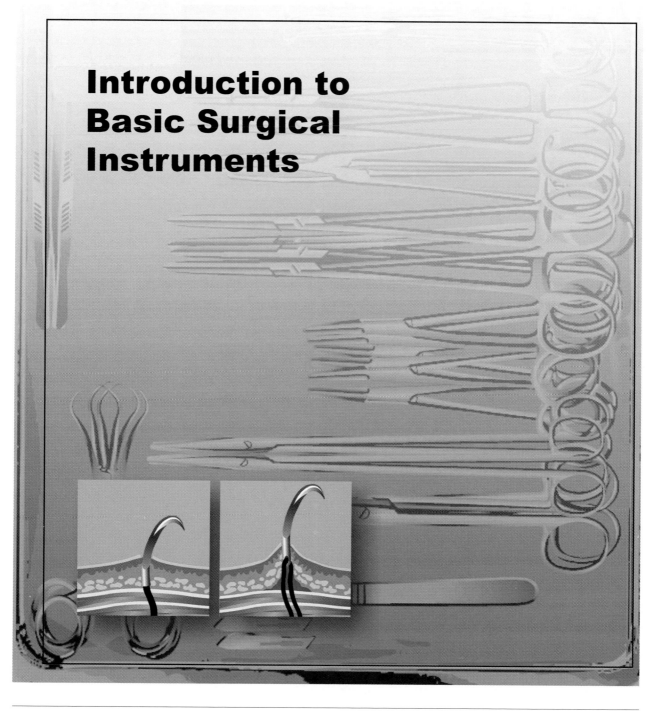

Chapter 1	Contents	Page

Surgical instruments have prehistoric roots in Indian, Chinese, Babylonian, Egyptian, and Roman civilizations. Today, hundreds of surgical instruments are used for specific functions or are designed to serve a common task. The aim of this chapter is to introduce basic surgical instruments that are used for common surgical procedures.

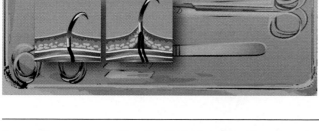

1:1 Scalpel

A scalpel is used for division of tissue and consists of a blade and handle (Figure 1.1). Although some scalpels are made of one solid piece of steel that includes both the handle and the blade, the majority of scalpels have a separate handle and a removable blade. Blades are available in a variety of shapes, each designed for a specific purpose. The most common blades have a straight back and an oval shaped sharp cutting front (Figure 1.2).

The most commonly used blade sizes are #10, #20, #21 and #22 (Figure 1.2). Figure 1.3 demonstrates other designs of scalpel blades which include a bayonet tip blade #11(a), a bistoury blade #12(b), and a small blade #15(c). Handle #4 fits into larger blades (#'s 20, 21, 22, 25) (Figure 1.2) and handles #3, 7, and 9 fit into smaller blades (#'s 10, 11, 12, 15) (Figure 1.3).

1:2 Scissors

Scissors are used for cutting, dissecting and debriding tissue. They may also be used for cutting sutures, bandages, and dressings. Scissors can either be long or short, and/or with blades that are straight or curved. Their tips can be both sharp, one sharp and one blunt, or both blunt (Figure 1.4). Mayo (Figure 1.5) and Metzenbaum (Figure 1.6) scissors are two basic types of scissors for tissue dissection. Metzenbaum scissors (or "mets") are the favourite among surgeons as they are lighter and longer instruments with a gentle curve near the end. Figure 1.7 demonstrates bandage scissors.

NB: Mayo scissors are used for heavy, hard and thick tissue as well as sutures, gauze, tubes, etc. Metzenbaum scissors, on the other hand, are used for tissue dissection and fine work only. Do not cut sutures or other materials with mets.

notes...

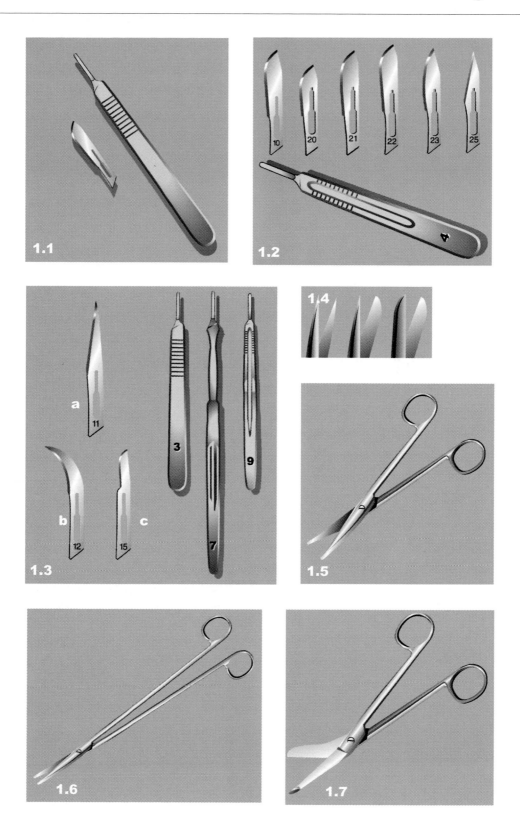

1:3 Sutures

A suture is a strand of material used to ligate (tie) blood vessels or approximate (sew) tissues. The use of plant strings or animal sinews for wound closure was described by many ancient civilizations (e.g. Chinese, Babylonians, Greeks). In the past, many materials have been used for this purpose: dried gut, dried tendon, strips of hide, horsehair, human hair, bark fibres, etc. The word "suture" is commonly used to refer to a suture with a needle for sewing, whereas a suture without a needle, used for tying, is referred to as a "tie". The tie may either be "free", referring to a straight strand of suture material, or on a "reel", where the suture is on a spool for multiple ligatures.

Suture materials can be classified by:

a) structure - monofilament and multifilament.
b) behaviour in tissue - absorbable and non-absorbable.
c) origin - organic, synthetic or metallic (Table 1).

notes...

Table 1 - Classification of Suture Materials

Note: Sutures are grouped according to their general characteristics. Some specific characteristics may not be noted.

Absorbable		Non-absorbable	
Name	Origin & characteristics	Name	Origin & characteristics
SURGIGUT® plain surgical gut	- collagen derived from submucosa of sheep intestine - soft yellowish or blue dyed - last within 7-10 days - digested by body enzymes	stainless surgical steel	- made of an alloy of iron-nickel and chromium - can be mono or multi filament - remains in the body indefinitely - non-reactive
SURGIGUT® chromic surgical gut	- same as plain gut but treated with chromium or aldehyde to resist digestion and increase durability in the body - loss of strength within 1 month - digested in 3 months	SOFSILK® silk	- braided natural fibers - looses strength in about 1 year, in 2 years cannot be found
POLYSORB® DEXON®	- polyglycolic acid. - strength decreased in one week and total absorption (hydrolized) in three months - colour is green	cotton	- twisted natural fibers - looses 50% of strength in 6 months, encapsulates in the body - seldom used
POLYSORB® VICRYL®	- coated, braided, synthetic - polyglycolic acid and polylactic acid - similar characteristics to chromic gut and Dexon® - colour is violet	BRALON® MONOSOFT® nylon	- coated, braided - monofilament - made of polyamide polymer - looses strength at a rate of 15-20% per year
BIOSYN® DEXON "S"® PDS® MAXON®	- polymer of polydioxanone - retains strength longer and remains longer in the body - colour is violet - same as Dexon® but smoother due to coating - polydioxanone monofilament - colour is violet - loss of strength within 90 days - modified polyglycolic acid - retains strength longer and remains longer in the body	SURGIDAC® SURGILINE® DACRON® MERSLINE® ETHIBOND® SURGIDAC® PROLENE® (poly-propylene) SURGIPRO® NOVAFIL®	- uncoated, monofilament, polyester - made of polyolefine - these are made from polyester-synthetic material that stays in the body indefinitely - coated, braided, polyester - made of a polyester propylene-synthetic material - stays in the body indefinitely - monofilament polypropylene - polybutester-synthetic - non-absorbable

a) Structure

i. Monofilament sutures (Figure 1.8) are made of a single strand of material and therefore encounter less resistance than multifilament sutures when passing through tissue . They also resist harbouring organisms which may cause suture tie infection. Monofilament sutures must be handled with care as crushing or crimping of the suture can nick or create a weak spot in the strand which may result in suture breakage.

ii. Multifilament sutures (Figure 1.9) consist of several filaments rendered into a strand by spinning, twisting or braiding. This provides greater tensile strength and pliability, but multifilament sutures can harbour infectious organisms between strands.

b) Behaviour in Tissue

i. Absorbable sutures are made from the collagen of healthy mammals (e.g. catgut) or from synthetic polymers (e.g. polyglycolic acid). They are used for temporary tissue approximation until sufficient wound healing has occurred to withstand normal stress. One major difference between the materials is that knots from synthetic material are more likely to slip than knots tied with biologic suture material. Organic (natural) absorbable sutures are absorbed into tissue after digestion by proteolytic enzymes, whereas synthetic absorbable sutures are hydrolyzed when water gradually penetrates the suture filaments and breaks down the polymer. Absorbable sutures may be organic (e.g. catgut) or synthetic (e.g. polyglycolic acid) (Table 1). Catgut (Figure 1.10) is made from the submucosa of sheep intestine or the serosa of bovine intestine and is 98% collagen. Plain catgut maintains tensile strength for only 7-10 days and is completely absorbed within 70 days.

In the second half of the 19th century, Lister treated catgut with chrome in order to prolong its life in vivo. The life of chromic catgut is about 3 months (90 days). The chromizing process alters the coloration of the surgical gut from yellowish-tan to brown (Figure 1.11). Chromic gut sutures maintain tensile strength for 10-14 days and cause less tissue irritation than plain gut.

Synthetic absorbable materials are primarily made of polyglycolic acid and its modifications (Figure 1.12).

The most widely used synthetic absorbable materials are POLYSORB®, DEXON®, PDS®, VICRYL®, BIOSYN® and MAXON®. These materials are primarily monofilaments and are absorbed into the tissue in about 90 days. Approximately 65%

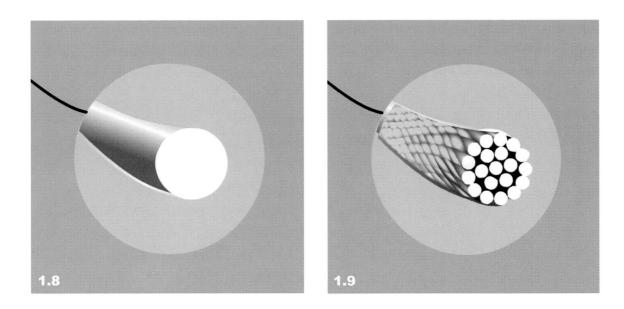

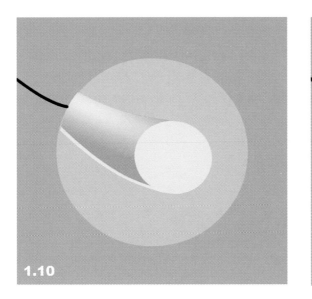
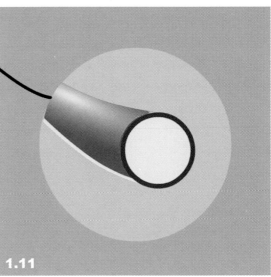

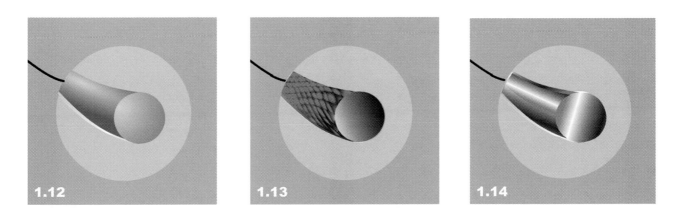

of original tensile strength is maintained at 14 days. Hydrolyzation of synthetic polymers causes less tissue reaction than enzymatic digestion of chrome. This is an important consideration in the surgeon's suture choice.

The most frequently used non-absorbable materials (Table 1) in surgery are silk, linen, cotton, and synthetic materials such as polyester (DACRON® O), polyamide (nylon), polyolefins (SURGIDAC®, SURGILENE®, PROLENE®) and polybutester (NOVA-FIL®, SURGIPRO®).

Silk is commonly used by surgeons (Figure 1.13) as it handles well and holds knots (i.e. does not slip). It is classified as non-absorbable, however in vivo studies have shown that it loses tensile strength in about one year and cannot usually be detected in tissue after 2 years. Therefore, in reality, silk is a very slow absorbing suture and hence should not be used in situations where long-term support of tissue is required (e.g. vascular grafts).

Metallic sutures, such as stainless steel and silver wire (Figure 1.14) are both commonly used in surgery today. Metallic sutures are indicated in areas of known infection and/or when it is desirable to avoid excessive tissue reaction. Other uses of metallic wire are in orthopaedic and plastic surgery repair of bones, ligaments and cartilage. Diameter of sutures can vary from 0.013 mm to 1.016 mm. The size of suture is directly related to the diameter of the thread. Size 0 is about .5 mm thick. When the diameter of the thread is smaller than 0.5, a "0" is added to the number, when it is larger, only the number is displayed for the size of suture. For example, "2-0" is thinner than "1-0" and "7-0" is thinner than "6-0" but size "2" is thicker than size "1". For a more detailed description of size and diameter see Table 2.

Table 2 - Metric Measures and USP Suture Diameter Equivalent

Organic Absorbable Materials		Non-absorbable and Synthetic Absorbable Materials	
USP Size Code	Suture Diameter (mm)	USP Size Code	Suture Diameter (mm)
8/0	0.05-0.069	8/0	0.038-0.051
7/0	0.07-0.099	7/0	0.051-0.076
6/0	0.10-0.14	6/0	0.076-0.102
5/0	0.15-0.19	5/0	0.102-0.152
4/0	0.20-0.24	4/0	0.152-0.203
3/0	0.25-0.29	3/0	0.203-0.254
2/0	0.30-0.39	2/0	0.254-0.330
0	0.40-0.49	0	0.330-0.406
1	0.50-0.59	1	0.406-0.483
2	0.60-0.69	2	0.483-0.559
3	0.70-0.79	3	0.559-0.635
4	0.80-0.89	4	0.635-0.711
5	0.90-0.99	5	0.711-0.813
6	1.00-1.09	6	0.813-0.914
		7	0.914-1.016

Table 3 - Suture Guide

Anatomical features	Suture type		Suture thickness	Needle type
	Absorbable	Non-abs		
A. Laparotomy				
• skin		•	4-0/3-0	Cutting
• subcuticular	•	•	5-0/3-0	Cutting
• subcutaneous fat	•		4-0/2-0	Taper
• fascia	•	•	2-0/1	Taper
• peritoneum	•		0	Taper
Inguinal ligament		•	2-0/1	Taper
Purse-string		•	4-0	Taper
Bowel Anastamosis				
• extended layer		•	4-0/2-0	Taper
• internal layer	•		4-0/2-0	Taper
B. Thoractomy				
• ribs		•	2-0/2	Taper
• periosteum		•	2-0/2	Taper
• skin & subcutaneous	same as abdominal wall			
• pleura		•	4-0	Taper
C. Cardiovascular surgery				
• pericardial retraction		•	2-0	Taper
• purse-string		•	2-0/4-0	Taper
• distal anastamosis		•	6-0/7-0	Taper
• proximal anastamosis		•	5-0/6-0	Taper
• aortic valve replacement		•± pledgets	2-0/3-0	Taper
• aortotomy closure		•	4-0	Taper
• mitral valve replacement		•± pledgets	2-0/0	Taper
• atrium closure		•	4-0/3-0	Taper
• vascular grafts		•	4-0/6-0	Taper
D. Urology				
• bladder tractions	•		2-0/0	Taper
• bladder closures		•	0/2	Taper
• ureter	•		4-0	Taper
• scrotum fascia	•		7-0/5-0	
• scrotum incision	•		5-0	Cutting
E. Plastic surgery				
• split thickness graft	•	•	6-0/4-0	Cutting
• full thickness graft		•	5-0/4-0	Cutting
• pedicle / flap graft	•	•	6-0	Cutting
• free flap graft				
-blood vessels		•	7-0	Taper
-edges of the flap		•	3-0/5-0	Cutting
• blepharoplasty	•	•	6-0/70	Cutting
• rhytidectomy		•	6-0/4-0	Cutting
• mammoplasty	•	•	3-0/5-0	Cutting
• tenoplasty / tenorrhaphy		•	4-0/6-0	Taper
F. Neurosurgery				
• dura		•	4-0/5-0	Taper
• galen		•	3-0	Cutting
• spinal cord dura				
-traction		•	2-0	Taper
-closures		•	5-0/3-0	Taper
-muscles, fascia	•		4-0	Cutting
-skin		•	5-0/4-0	Cutting

1:4 Needles

The surgical needle is as important as the suture. A surgical needle can be divided into three parts (Figure 1.15): the point, the body, and the tail or suture attachment end. The point is the sharp end of a needle, which can have a variety of shapes and configurations. The most widely used needle points are called "taper" and "cutting". The taper needle point (Figure 1.16 a) is round and is designed for soft tissue such as bowels or blood vessels. The body of the needle and the thread follow the tapered point and seal the hole made by the needle. This prevents bleeding or evacuation of microbes through the walls of contaminated cavities such as bowels.

The cutting needle point (Figure 1.16 b) has at least two, and often three, opposing cutting edges. These sharp edges enable the needle to go through tough tissue, such as skin, by cutting it. The cutting needle is used for hard tissue such as skin or fascia where the cutting of tissue does not create a danger for infection, bleeding or other complications.

The body of the needle may have different shapes. It can be 1/2, 3/8, 5/8, 1/4 of a circle or straight (Figure 1.17).

The tail of the needle has either an eye for the suture to be loaded or is swaged (atraumatic or "eyeless") (Figure 1.18). Needle eyes have various configurations. Eyed needles were often used in the past but are uncommon today. The disadvantage of an eyed needle is the double thread that follows the needle and traumatizes the tissue (Figure 1.19a). The advantage of atraumatic needles is that a single thread follows the needle and does not cause tearing of the tissue (Figure 1.19b).

NB: Absorbable sutures are not to be used on arteries, veins or places where high pressure or longer healing time is required. The size of the suture must always be matched to the thickness of the tissue. Cutting needles are not to be used on arteries, veins, guts or other organs where the possibility of bleeding or infection is evident after the closure.

notes...

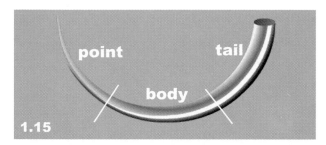

point   tail

body

1.15

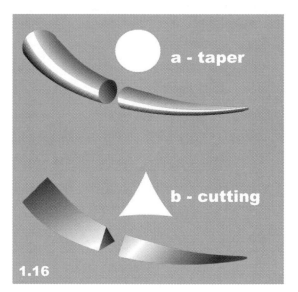

a - taper

b - cutting

1.16

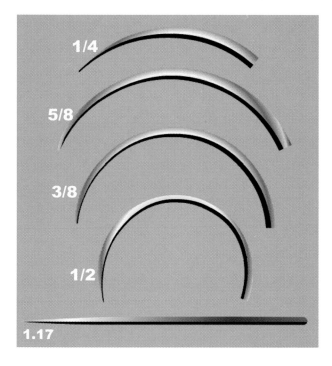

1/4

5/8

3/8

1/2

1.17

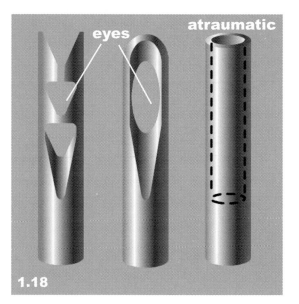

eyes   atraumatic

1.18

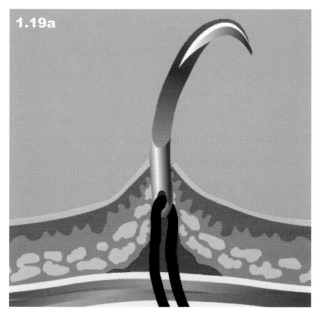

1.19a

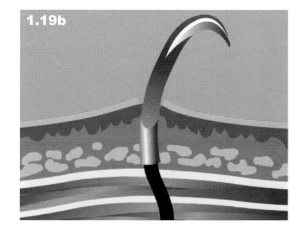

1.19b

1:5 Needle Holders

A needle holder (driver) is a surgical instrument that provides a firm grasp for a needle to be manipulated at a distance from the suture target. Needle holders have a variety of jaws and handles. The most commonly used needle holder has rings on the end of the handle (like scissors), a short blade jaw to hold the needle, and usually a locking mechanism (ratchet) (Figure 1.20).

The second type, or Castroviejo needle holder (Figure 1.21), does not have rings but instead consists of two strips of metal joined at one end with locking devices between them.

The jaws of a needle holder have a variety of configurations designed to provide a firm grip on different sized needles (Figure 1.22).

NB: The size of the needle must always match the size of the needle holder.

notes...

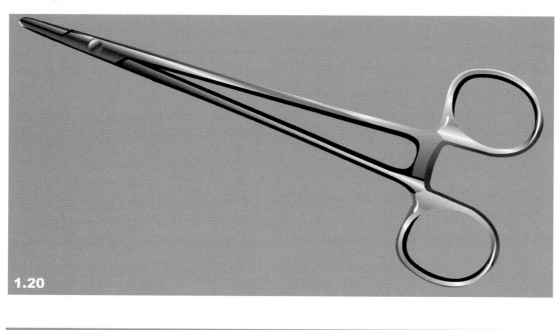

1.20

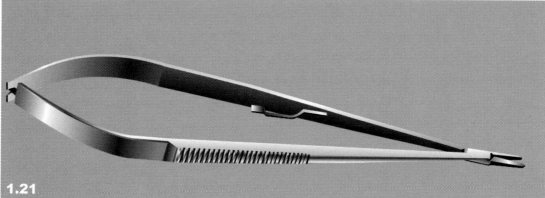

1.21

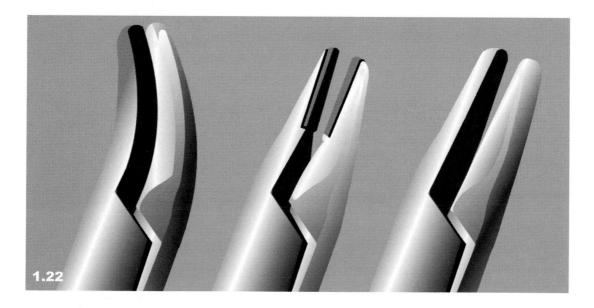

1.22

1:6 Forceps

The word "forceps" describes different types of surgical instruments:
a) thumb forceps
b) grasping forceps
c) hemostatic forceps
d) other types of forceps

a) Thumb forceps consist of two strips of metal joined at one end and are used to pick up tissue or hold tissue between opposed surfaces (Figure 1.23), thereby giving a surgeon more control over the amount of pressure applied to the tissue. The needle "tips" or "heads" on the opposing surfaces of forceps create a variety of designs specific to the use of the instrument:.

i) if the tips are blunt, the instrument is called a dressing forceps (Figure 1.24a).

ii) if the branches have teeth, or are serrated, it is called a tissue forceps (Figure 1.24b).

iii) if the branches are sharp, it is called a splinter forceps (Figure 1.24c).

b) Grasping forceps are designed to hold tissues strong enough to allow one to exert traction. The opposing heads vary depending on the instrument's specific purpose. All have a set or finger grip, and a locking mechanism.

i) Debaky forceps are a special type of forceps that have a flat end point covered with fine teeth and a longitudinal groove (Figure 1.25).

ii) Figure 1.26 demonstrates a Babcock clamp (forceps) used for grasping delicate tissue and tubular structures, e.g. vermiform appendix or fallopian tube. This instrument has curved empty triangular branches and the base of each triangle opposes one another.

iii) The Allis clamp (forceps) has opposing serrated tips with short teeth used for grasping tough tissues such as fascia (Figure 1.27).

iv) A Kocher clamp (forceps) has short transverse serrations along the length of the blades and the tips have sharp teeth (Figure 1.28).

NB: Hard clamps with teeth are not to be used on viable tissue as they are designed to crush the tissue.

notes...

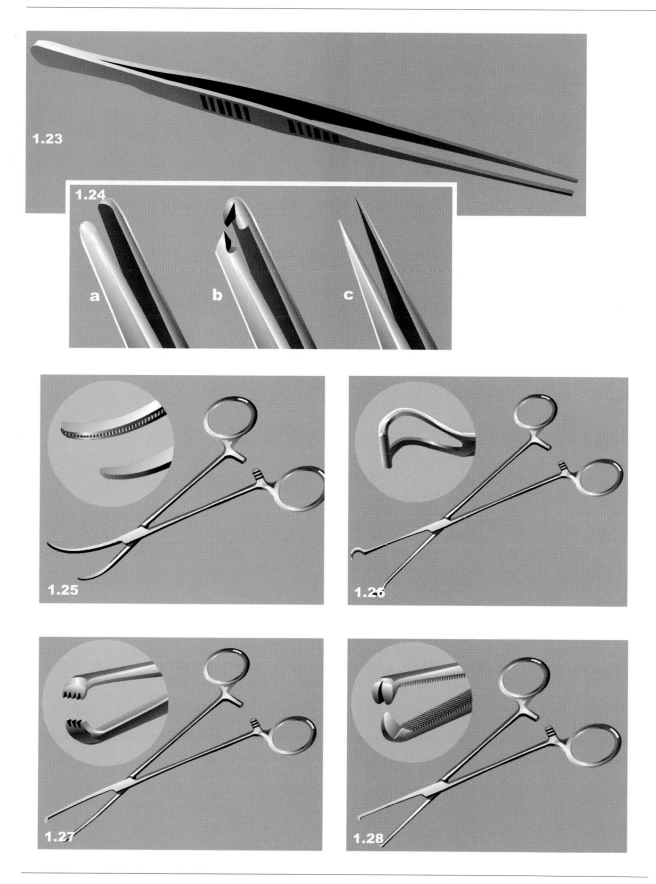

c) Hemostatic forceps or clamps look similar to needle holders and grasping forceps since they all have a pair of finger rings and a locking mechanism. Hemostatic clamps (forceps) can have straight or curved blades (Figure 1.29). They can be hard and forceful and able to crush tissue (crushing) or they can be soft in order to stop bleeding and not crush tissue (non-crushing).

i) Hard clamps. The most frequently used hemostatic clamps are called "snaps" or "Criles". Other types include: "mosquitoes" which are light and small (Figure 1.30 a); heavy arterial clamps (Kelly) (Figure 1.30 b); and Lauer clamps (right angle) (Figure 1.31) that have an entirely curved tip. Mosquitoes and Kellies are used for permanent hemostasis of the bleeding points, with subsequent ligation of the bleeding vessel.

ii) Soft clamps. These are used to temporarily interrupt blood flow in a blood vessel. Figure 1.32a demonstrates a clamp used for major vessels such as the aorta. Figure 1.32b shows a soft "bulldog" clamp used for medium-sized blood vessels. Hemorrhoidal or lung clamps (Figure 1.33) have triangular tips with serrated surfaces. They have strong grasping power and allow significant traction to be applied. These are commonly used on heavy fascia.

d) Other types of forceps. These include towel clips or towel-holding forceps with two sharp or flat ends which hold the edges of a towel in place (Figures 1.34a & 1.34b). Sponge holding clamps (Figure 1.35) have large rings with serrated surfaces.

NB: Hard hemostatic clamps on a major artery or vein damage the endothelium and may cause calcification with subsequent occlusion of the artery. Therefore, only soft clamps are used for temporary hemostasis on major blood vessels.

notes...

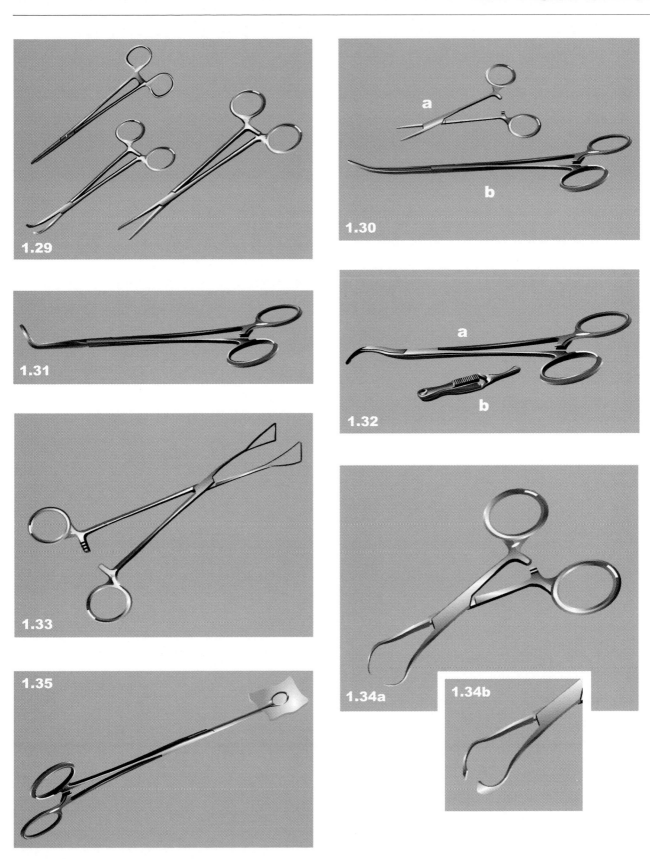

1.29

1.30

1.31

1.32

1.33

1.34a

1.34b

1.35

1:7 Retractors

Retractors are surgical instruments that are used to improve the visibility of the operating field by holding the tissue aside. There are many types of retractors. Those most commonly used are presented in Figure 1.36.

Figure 1.37 represents a plain retractor that has simple strips of metal fashioned into curves at each end (Parker).

Rake retractors (Figure 1.38) have curved, blunt or sharp tips, and are commonly used for retracting skin edges.

Self-retaining retractors (Figure 1.39) have a simple locking mechanism that holds the retractor and the wound open without someone holding it.

Figure 1.40 demonstrates a surgical tray with additional instruments used for simple surgical procedures.

NB: Success of a surgical procedure may depend on good exposure. Retractors expose the operating field and can be added and/or replaced to explore the depth in separate planes. Sharp retractors with teeth should not be used where organs can be perforated.

notes...

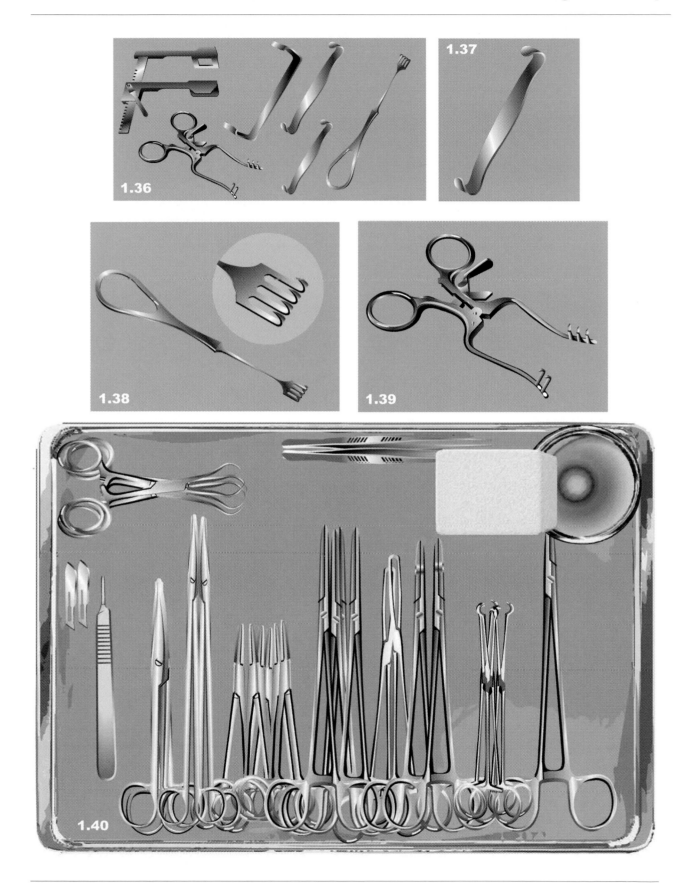

Chapter 2

Handling of
Surgical Instruments

Chapter 2	Contents	Page

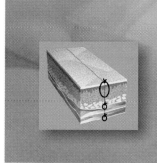

The use of surgical instruments for specific tasks may require skills that positively affect the outcome of a surgical procedure. These skills include holding, handling and maneuvering surgical instruments in such a way that makes the performance of the surgical procedure safer, easier, smoother, and faster. It is important to mention that there are no specific rules and regulations for the holding and handling of surgical instruments. Individual surgeons may develop their own style of operating. Therefore, it is feasible to select specific maneuvers from different operators and form a style that one is most comfortable with. The specific aim of this chapter is to introduce the most commonly used (classic) methods for holding, handling and maneuvering surgical instruments during operating procedures.

2:1 Operating the Scalpel

2:1:1 Handling a Scalpel

A scalpel is a sharp instrument and therefore it is important to use *extreme caution* when handling. In terms of handling sharp objects in the operating room, treat every patient as though they have a blood-borne transmissible disease.

a) Loading. Loading and unloading of the blade must be done with a hemostatic clamp or needle driver by grasping the body of the blade and sliding the blade onto the hub of the handle (Figure 2.1).

b) Unloading. To unload the scalpel, grasp the proximal end of the blade with a hemostatic clamp, push the blade slightly upward to unlock the body of the blade, and separate the blade from the handle by sliding the blade upward (Figure 2.2).

c) Giving. To give the scalpel to another person, the scalpel should be grasped with the sharp edge of the blade downward, the head toward the person who is giving the scalpel and the handle toward the person who is receiving the scalpel (Figure 2.3).

d) Receiving. To receive the scalpel, grasp the handle and move the scalpel down and then toward yourself (Figure 2.4).

NB: A scalpel is a sharp instrument, hence:
The scalpel must not be loaded and unloaded manually - use instruments.
The scalpel must never be passed to others with the sharp end toward the receiver as it may injure the receiving individual.
When receiving the scalpel, do not pull the scalpel as it may cut the fingers of the other person.

notes...

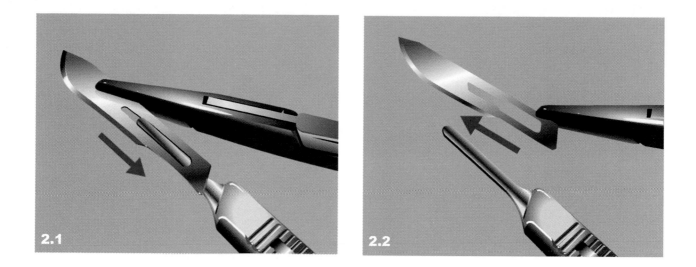

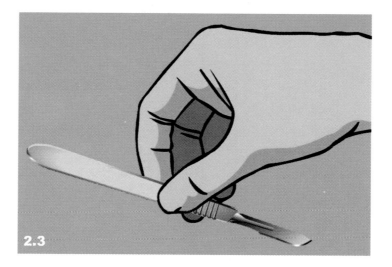

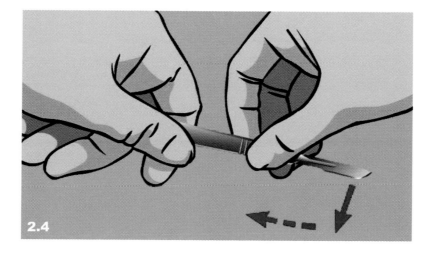

2:1:2 Holding a Scalpel

The most important principle to remember when holding a scalpel is to have full control of the instrument and at the same time, to have freedom of movement. There are three common ways to hold a scalpel:

a) The Pencil Grip (Figure 2.5). This grip is used to perform small, precise incisions often with a #15 blade. With this grip, the cutting direction can be changed 360° by moving the hand and wrist (with little upper arm movement).

b) The Fingertip Grip (Figure 2.6). This grip is used to make long, straight, or curved incisions. This technique provides a great deal of maneuverability due to the flexibility of the arm, wrist and fingers. As a result, it is frequently used in surgery.

c) The Palm Grip (Figure 2.7). This is the strongest grip and used when a precise movement with a great deal of pressure is required. The hand and wrist are kept relatively fixed, and the scalpel is held parallel with the skin to maximize the cutting edge of the blade. This grip has very limited maneuverability.

notes...

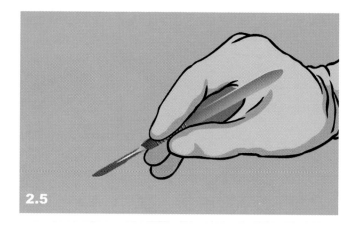

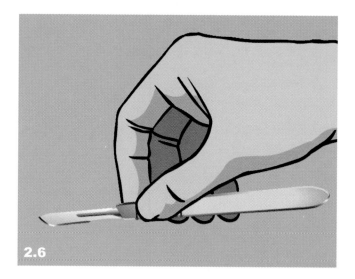

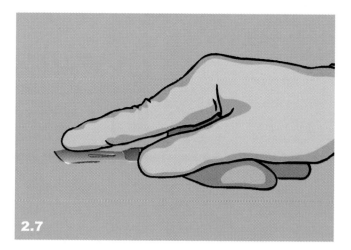

2:1:3 Incision Techniques

General Principles:

The most important principles for the use of the scalpel are as follows:

a) planning and measuring before cutting.

b) stabilizing the skin during an incision (Figure 2.8).

c) placing the knife perpendicular to the tissue plane and cutting straight and clean (Figure 2.9).

d) cutting the tissue layer by layer.

e) focusing your attention on the direction of the scalpel when cutting.

Methods:

The most common methods of incision with a scalpel are:

a) Press Cutting. The scalpel is pressed into the depth of the tissue with a straight movement, like stabbing (Figure 2.10).

b) Slide Cutting. The sharp edge of the blade slides on the surface of the tissue with a specific pressure and depth (Figure 2.11).

c) Sawing. The cutting is performed by sliding the sharp edge of the blade with push-pull movements, like sawing a log (Figure 2.12).

d) Scraping. The scalpel blade is held at an acute angle to the tissue surface to be scraped and used with a side-sliding motion on the surface of the tissue, similar to shaving whiskers with a straight razor blade (Figure 2.13).

notes...

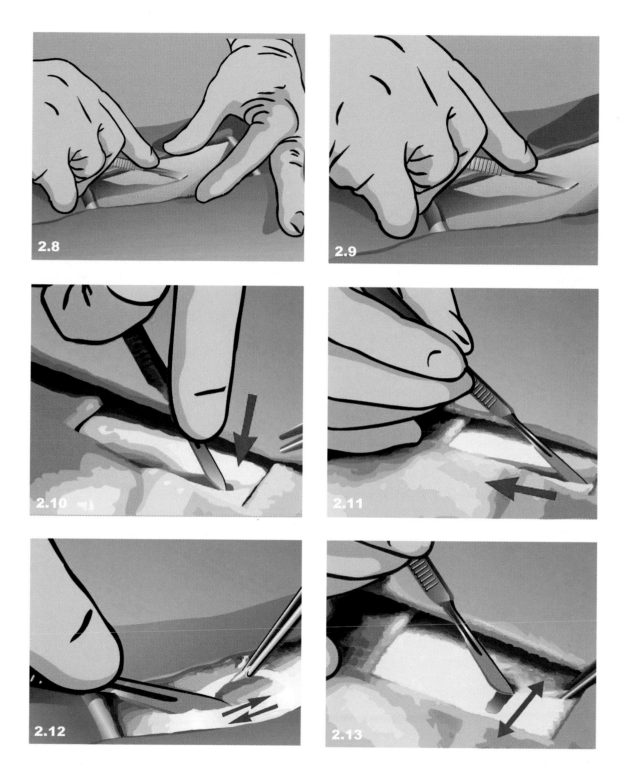

2.8

2.9

2.10

2.11

2.12

2.13

Operating Scissors

2:2:1 Holding Scissors

The most common ways to hold scissors are as follows:

a) Thumb-Ring Finger Grip. The thumb and ring fingers are inserted into the scissor rings, the middle finger is rested in front and on top of the ring finger, and the index finger is placed on the shanks (Figure 2.14 a and b). This is the most common grip for precise cutting of the tissue and for maximum control.

b) Thumb-Index Finger Grip. In this grip, the thumb and the index finger are placed into the rings and the body of the scissors is placed in the palm of the hand (Figure 2.15). This grip is used for direction control in reverse cutting or for deep body cavities such as the chest.

c) One Finger Grip. The scissors are held by one finger in one ring (Figure 2.16) and no finger in the other ring. This method does not provide a good grip and is rarely used.

d) No Finger Grip. The scissors are held with no fingers in the rings (Figure 2.17). This grip is primarily for using right-handed scissors with the left hand, and has very limited use.

2:2:2 Using Scissors

General Principles:

The most important principles for using scissors are:

a) Use the most comfortable grip that provides the best stability for direction control.

b) Do not push the fingers far into the ring. Use only the tips of the fingers to operate the scissors and use the tips of the scissors for cutting.

c) Control hemostasis before cutting.

d) Always measure and think before cutting.

e) When cutting sutures, secure a good position in order to see both the suture to be divided and the tips of the scissors. This will prevent cutting other structures.

f) When bringing scissors into the surgical field or approaching a suture to be cut, keep the tips closed, open and cut, then retrieve. Do not "dive-bomb" into the field with the jaws wide open.

g) Ensure that the suture is cut before withdrawing the scissors otherwise traction may be put on an incompletely cut suture which may disrupt the vessel being ligated.

h) Squeeze the blades of the scissors together so that the sharp edges "grind" together as they cut (especially for thick sutures such as "0" or larger).

Movement :

Three types of movements can be made with scissors: closing, torque and shearing. With these three forces, it is possible to chew-cut, crush-cut, or push-cut the tissue. Scissors can also be used for blunt dissection.

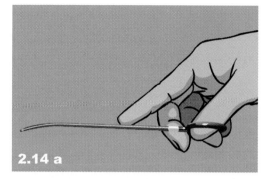

2.14 a

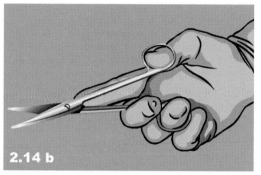

2.14 b

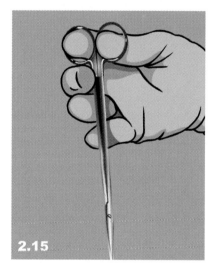

2.15

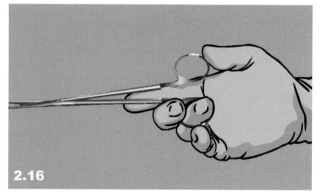

2.16

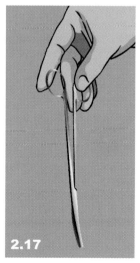

2.17

2:3 Operating a Needle Holder

2:3:1 Holding Needle Holders

Four types of grips are commonly used for needle holders:

a) Thumb-Ring-Finger Grip (Figure 2.18) is the same as described for scissors.

b) Palm Grip (Figure 2.19) is the strongest grip used in places where it is difficult to advance the needle.

c) Ring-Finger Grip (Figure 2.20) is when the needle holder is in the palm of the hand with only the ring finger in one of the rings.

d) Pencil Grip (Figure 2.21) is used with Castrovajo type needle holders

2:3:2 Loading a Needle Holder with a Needle

The relationship of the needle and the needle holder jaw is important to mention in this chapter due to frequent problems, such as bending the needle, which can happen when the needle is held by the needle holder too far back near the tail. Excessive torque on the needle, instead of driving the needle with pronation and supination of the wrist, results in the bending and breaking of the needle.

In special circumstances, the needle holder can be placed close to the point at the front of the needle, in the middle of the needle body or close to the tail of the needle, as required. However, one of the most commonly used methods is to visually divide the needle into three parts and place the jaw of the needle holder onto the border between the middle third and the tail of the needle (Figure 2.22). This position leaves sufficient length for the needle to pass through the thickness of the tissue while preventing it from bending and deformation. The tail of the needle is the weakest part of the needle.

Needles can be placed with different angles in relation to the needle holder, i.e. perpendicular to the holder (right angle, Figure 2.22) or at a wide (Figure 2.23 a) or sharp (Figure 2.23 b) angle "hooking the needle".

NB: The angle of the needle with respect to the needle holder should be chosen in such a way to make the needle perpendicular to the line of sewing. In other words, the angle of the needle should be related to the position of the operator.

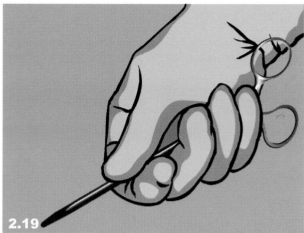

2.18

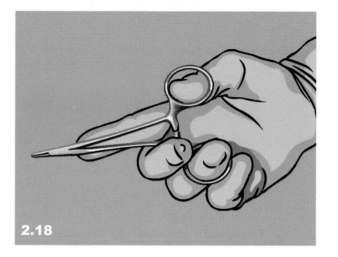

2.19

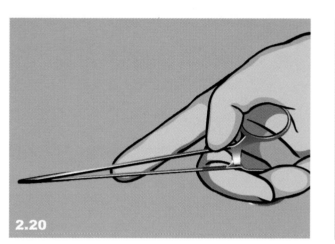

2.20

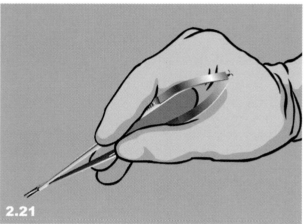

2.21

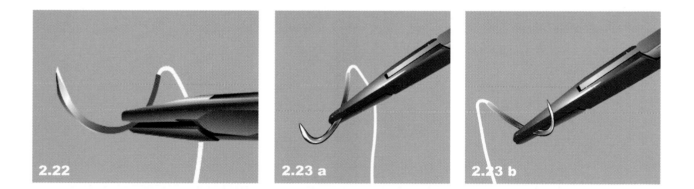

2.22

2.23 a

2.23 b

General Principles:

The most important principles in operating a needle holder are:

a) Avoidance of Stuttering. Stuttering describes the non-productive repetition of steps needed to be done only once. This occurs most often before the needle is in the tissue.

b) Avoidance of Stammering. Stammering is described as an interruption during a step that could be done with one motion and usually occurs after the needle is inserted into the tissue.

c) A forehand stitch should be started from the far side of the wound and sewn toward oneself (Figure 2.24).

d) A backhand stitch starts from the near side and finishes at the far side; the needle is loaded backwards (Figure 2.25).

e) The needle should be placed perpendicular to the tissue plane. The driving force is always in the direction of the segment of a needle within the tissue. The rotating force must be non-stressful and done with the rotation of the wrist (Figure 2.26 a and b).

f) The far side of the wound should be grasped gently by forceps and everted outward to expose both the under layers and the needle entrance in the wound (Figure 2.27).

g) On the near side of the wound, the target layer is grasped by the forceps and the needle pushed through. In order to see the needle exit, grasp the upper layers and retract them away from oneself.

h) When sewing is complete, keep the sharp end of the needle backward and parallel to the needle holder (Figure 2.28).

i) Tissue should be sewn layer by layer and each layer should be identified (Figure 2.29).

notes...

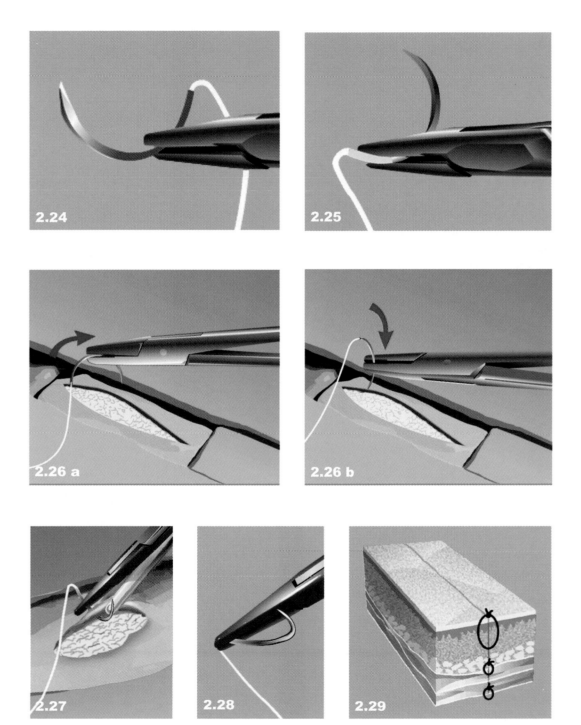

2:4 Operating Tissue Forceps

2:4:1 Holding Tissue Forceps

The best way to grip tissue forceps is to hold the forceps between the fingers in such a position that the thumb is on one blade and the index finger and third finger are on the opposite blade (Figure 2.30). This position, with the thumb against the index finger (metacarpophalangeal joint), gives the widest range of flexibility to maneuver the tissue forceps. When the tissue forceps are not in use, they should be held in the palm of the hand and secured with the little finger or ring finger (Figure 2.31). Figure 2.32 demonstrates an undesirable hold that restricts the maneuverability of the operator on all planes.

2:4:2 Using Tissue Forceps

Forceps are used for a variety of reasons in a surgical procedures such as holding tissue during cutting, retracting for exposure, stabilizing during suturing, extracting needles, grasping vessels for cautery, passing ligatures around hemostats, packing sponges, or everting skin edges for clipping.

General Principles:

The most important principles for the proper handling of tissue forceps include:

a) Never keep inactive forceps in the palm of the hand as it restricts maneuverability.

b) When turning forceps from a passive position to an active position, hold the palm down as gravity aids the shift from a "hold" to a "use" position.

c) Do not keep elbows close to the body as this restricts mobility.

d) Do not crush and traumatize tissue with the forceps.

notes...

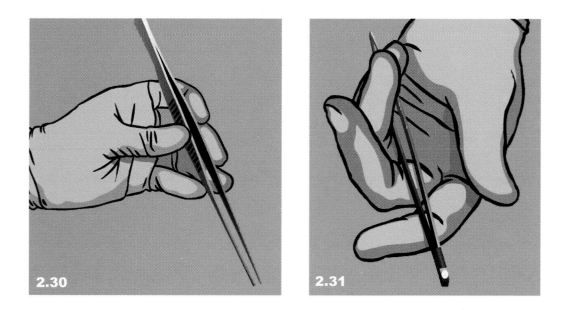

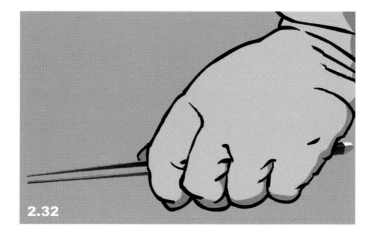

2:5 Operating Clamps

2:5:1 Holding a Surgical Clamp

a) Thumb and Ring Finger. A surgical clamp is usually held like a needle holder or scissors with the thumb in one ring, the ring finger in the other ring, the third finger over the top of the ring and the index finger on the junction of the branches (Figure 2.33).

b) Thumb and Index Finger. The surgical clamp can also be held by entering the thumb into one ring, the index finger into the second ring, the middle and ring fingers on the back of the second ring, and holding the clamp in the palm of the hand (Figure 2.34).

c) Multiple Holding. Sometimes multiple hemostatic clamps need to be applied. In this case, clamps are held in the palm and applied one by one (Figure 2.35 a).

d) Classical Clamp Removal. For clamp removal, use the same grip as with the application of the clamp and remove by squeezing the ring and thumb fingers, and keeping the locking mechanism apart while opening the jaws (Figure 2.35 b).

e) Other Techniques of Clamp Removal. Clamps can also be removed without hav-

ing the fingers in the rings (Figure 2.36). In this technique, the left ring is pinched between the thumb and ring finger and the lock is disengaged by pressing the index finger beneath the opposite ring of the clamp.

notes...

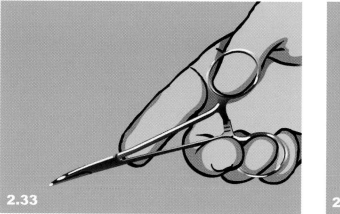

2.33

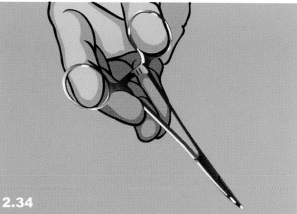

2.34

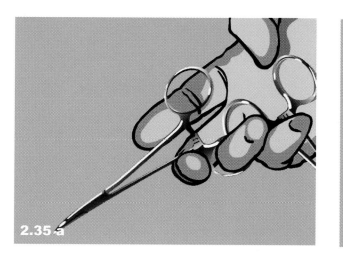

2.35 a

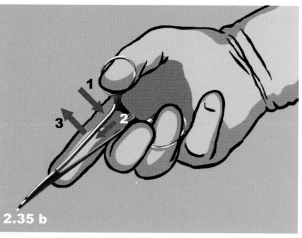

2.35 b

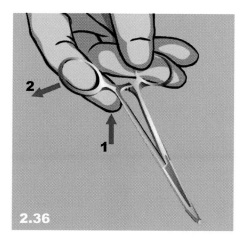

2.36

2:5:2 Using a Surgical Clamp

Surgical clamps can be used in many situations including hemostasis, dissection, retraction, holding the tissue, passing the ligature, and occlusion of tubular structures such as blood vessels, bowel or bronchioles. There are two methods to apply a hemostatic clamp:

a) Apply on the dissected blood vessel before bleeding begins. In this case, two hemostatic clamps are applied proximal and distal to the target area and the vessel is cut between the clamps (Figure 2.37).

b) Trapping the bleeding vessel in the convexity of its jaw (Figure 2.38).

Ligation of a clamp takes several steps:

a) Hold the clamp upward and away from the tissue (while the surgeon passes the ligature around the clamp (Figure 2.39).

b) Lower the clamp parallel to the tissue to expose the tip (for surgeon to pass the ligature around to encircle completely, (Figure 2.40).

c) Tilt the clamp slightly on its side in order to expose the side where the surgeon is tying the knot.

d) Slowly release the clamp as the surgeon tightens down the knot so that tissue does not slip before it is secured in the ligature.

e) For additional security, one may suture under the clamp. Circle the first half of the clamp, and then the other half, before tying (Figure 2.41a & b).

General Principles:

The most important principles for the application and removal of surgical clamps are:

a) It is always a two person job; it should not be done alone.

b) Before removing the clamp, make sure that the ligature is situated beneath the clamp.

c) Always remove the clamp slowly and with simultaneous tying of the ligature by a partner.

d) Never apply clamps blindly, clean the wound with sponges and/or suction in order to cause minimal trauma to the tissue.

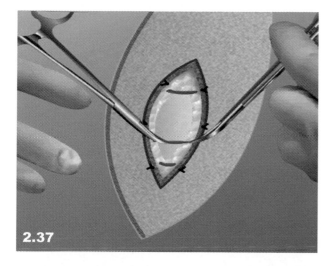

2.37

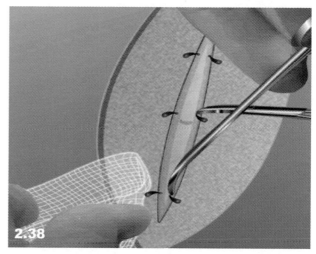

2.38

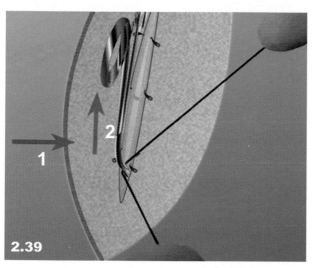

2.39

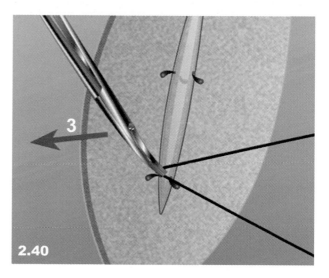

2.40

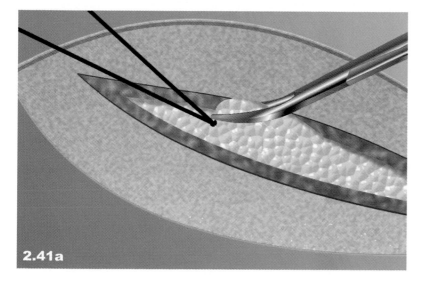

2.41a

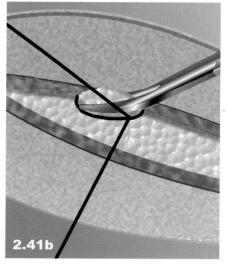

2.41b

Chapter 3

Knot Tying Techniques

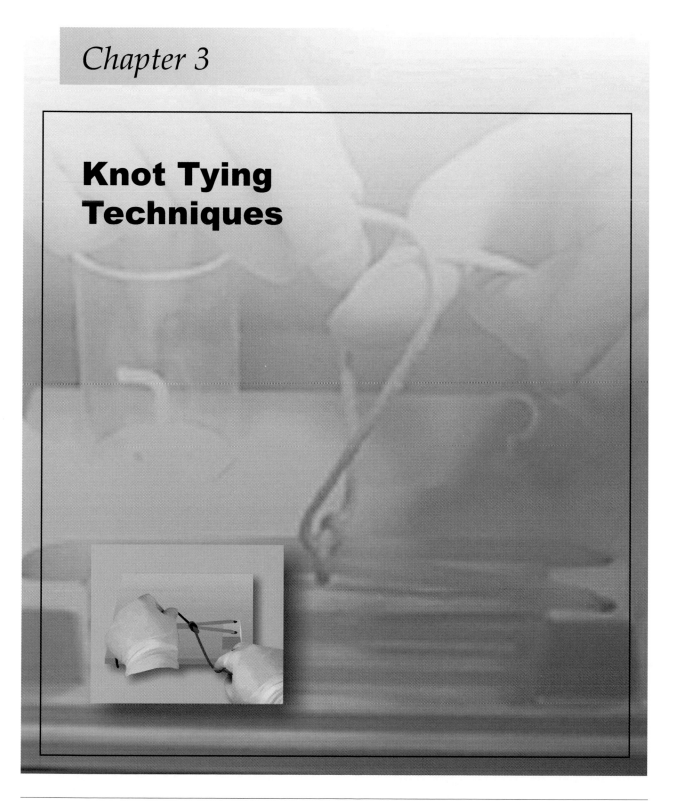

Chapter 3	Contents	Page

Knot tying techniques are the most basic, yet the most essential surgical skills. All that is required are the surgeons' hands and suture material. Hand-tied knots are applied in many tasks such as hemostasis, anastomosis between hollow organs (e.g. bowel or blood vessels), and wound closure. Therefore, it is important for a surgeon to master a variety of surgical knots and knot tying techniques. There are two important components of knot tying skills: quality and speed. High quality knots are square, tight and placed without trauma to the tissue. Quality and speed are inter-related and one should not be sacrificed for the other. Concentration should be placed first on tying quality knots, followed by practice to increase speed.

3:1 Types of Surgical knots

Surgeons generally use four basic knots:

a) Simple Knot. An incomplete, one unit knot (Figure 3.1).

b) Granny Knot. A two unit knot that is completed by repeating identical steps. It is a sliding knot (slips under pressure) and therefore should only be used for purposes such as approximation of high tension wounds (e.g. lateral thoracotomy) and should be completed with a third mirror-image knot that makes it square (Figure 3.2).

c) Square Knot. A two unit knot that is completed with two mirror-image simple knots. This is a very strong knot and is by far the knot most often used in surgery (Figure 3.3).

d) Surgeon's or Friction Knot. The first unit of this knot is a double loop and the second unit is a single loop mirror-image. It is used as a tension tie and is a very safe technique for beginners (Figure 3.4).

NB: It is always preferable to make three or more knots depending on the quality of material and size of the suture. Smaller sized sutures and synthetic materials need more knots. Generally, use three knots for silk, 4-5 knots for synthetic absorbable, and six knots for synthetic monofilament non-absorbable materials.

3:2 Tying Techniques

Techniques for tying a surgical knot can be divided into two-handed, one-handed and instrument tying. The suture is subdivided into two segments which are called the active and passive strands. The active strand is the segment of the suture that is manipulated and the passive strand is the one that is manipulated on. In a two-handed knot tying technique, the active strand is always the closest one to the operator and it should be kept in the right hand. After completion of the knot it should be pulled toward the assistant in order to make the knot flat. If the active strand is not in the right hand, the strands may cross when the loop is formed (Figure 3.5a). In this case, it is impossible to flatten and hence affects the quality of the knot. Figure 3.5b shows the correct configeration.

notes...

*For all diagrams, the active strand is red
and the passive strand is **black**.*

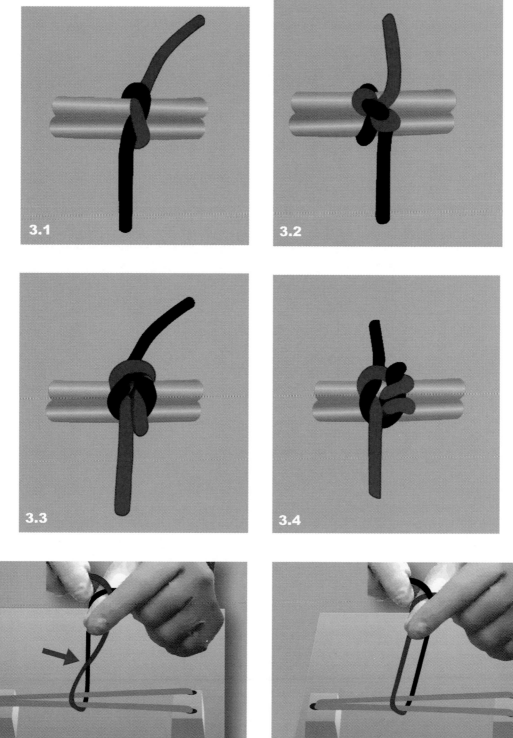

3:2:1 Two-Handed Ties

Grasp both segments of the thread with the middle, ring and little fingers and keep the index finger and the thumb free for manipulation (Figure 3.6).

Unit One - Active strand (red) toward the operator (for right handed people the active strand or segment is in the right hand).

a) Form a loop around the index finger by bringing the active strand over the top of the index finger (Figure 3.7).

b) Pinch the index finger and the thumb (Figure 3.8).

c) Swing the pinched index finger and the thumb from under the loop to the opposite side of the loop (Figure 3.9).

d) Throw the active strand over the loop and grasp it between the pinched index finger and thumb (Figure 3.10).

e) Pass the active strand through from under the loop (Figure 3.11).

f) Grasp the active thread from under the loop and put the knot down with the help of index finger (Figure 3.12).

notes...

*For all diagrams, the active strand is red and the passive strand is **black**.*

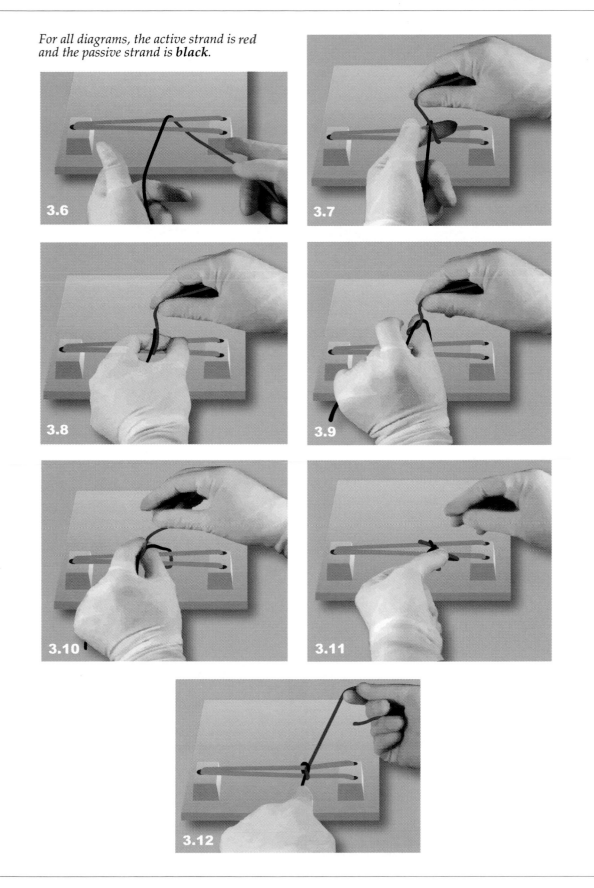

Unit Two - Active strand opposite the operator.

a) Move the left thumb inside the passive strand and form a loop around the thumb by bringing the active strand over the top of the thumb (Figure 3.13).

b) Pinch the thumb and the index finger together (Figure 3.14).

c) Swing the pinched thumb and index finger from under the loop to the opposite side and grasp the active strand (Figure 3.15).

d) Pass the active strand through the loop (Figure 3.16).

e) Grasp the active thread from under the loop and put the knot down with the help of index finger (Figure 3.17).

N.B.: In the two-handed tie, the left hand takes an active part in setting up the loop and manipulating the active strand for a right handed person. If only unit one is applied, it is a simple knot; if two identical units are applied, it is a granny knot; if both units one and two are applied, it is a square knot.

notes...

*For all diagrams, the active strand is red
and the passive strand is black.*

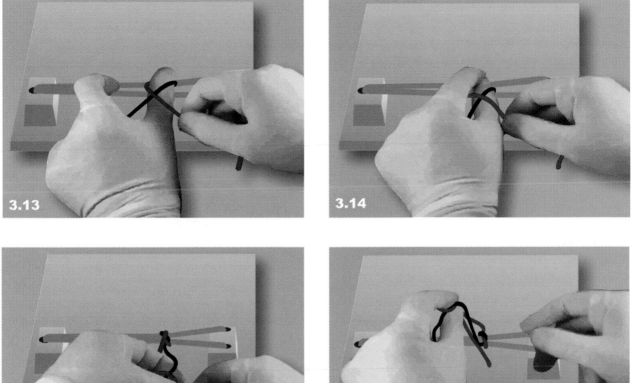

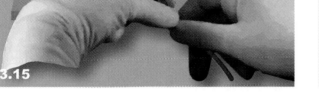

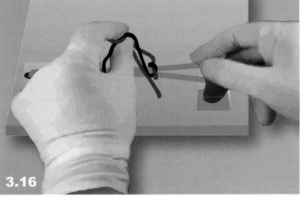

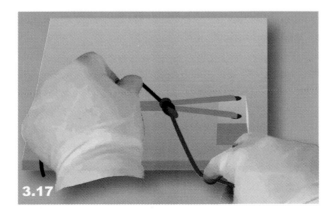

3:2:2 One-Handed Ties

Unit One - Active strand (red) toward the operator (if right-handed, the active strand is in the left hand).

a) For this knot, grasp the strands with thumb and index finger and leave the three fingers, namely middle, ring and little fingers free for manipulation (Figure 3.18).

b) Make a loop around three fingers with the passive (black) strand over the top. Keep the angle indicated in Figure 3.19 as wide as possible.

c) Flex the middle finger, hook the active (red) strand and grasp it between the middle and ring fingers (Figure 3.20).

d) Sweep the active (red) strand from under the loop by holding it between the middle and ring fingers (Figure 3.21).

e) Tighten the knot with the left index finger (Figure 3.22).

notes...

*For all diagrams, the active strand is red and the passive strand is **black**.*

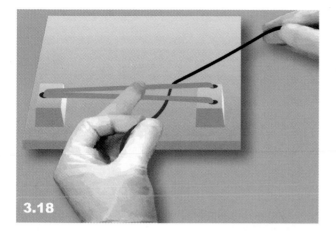

3.18

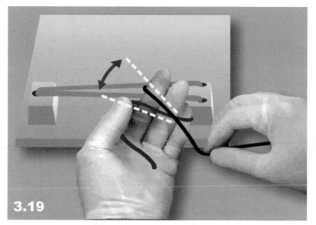

3.19

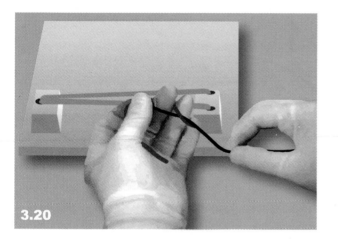

3.20

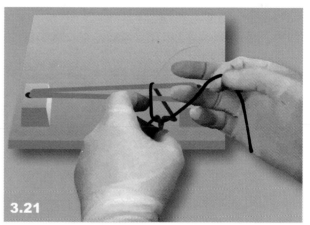

3.21

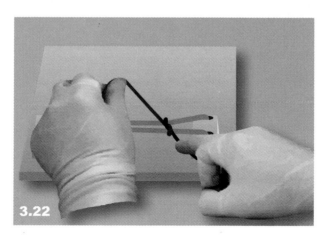

3.22

Unit Two - Active strand opposite the operator.

a) Grasp the active (red) strand with thumb and middle finger (Figure 3.23).

b) Make a loop around the index finger by moving the index finger under the active (red) strand and bringing the passive (black) over the top of the index finger (Figure 3.24).

c) Flex the left index finger catching the active (red) strand with the dorsum of the finger (fingernail) (Figure 3.25).

d) Sweep the active strand through the loop with the help of the index finger (Figure 3.26).

e) Grasp the active strand from under the loop with the same hand and tighten with the index finger (Figure 3.27).

N.B.: In the one-handed-tie, either the right or left hand can be used to set up the loop and manipulate the active strand. Therefore, with the one-handed technique, the square knot can be formed by applying two different units or using the same unit with both right and left hand.

notes...

For all diagrams, the active strand is **red**
and the passive strand is **black**.

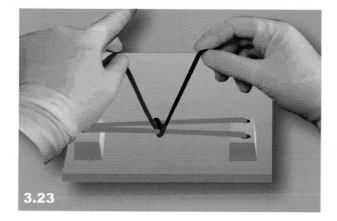

3.23

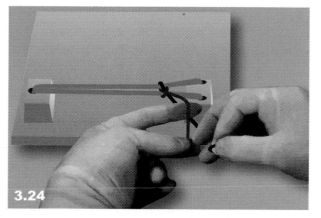

3.24

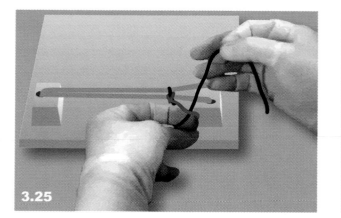

3.25

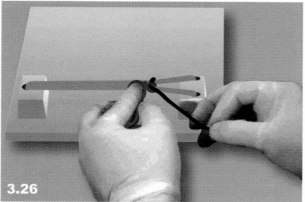

3.26

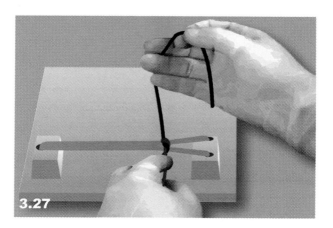

3.27

3:2:3 Surgeon's or Friction Knot

Sometimes it is challenging to keep the first knot in place while placing the second knot. The reasons may include the nature of the thread or the tensile strains pulling the wound in the opposite direction. In order to avoid loosening of the first knot, one of the strands should always be kept with a slight tension while the second knot is completed. Surgeon's or friction knots can also be used to keep the first knot in place during the placement of the second knot.

Steps:

a) Repeat unit one of the two-handed knot tying technique (Figures 3.28 - 3.32).

• Form a loop around the index finger.
• Pinch the index finger and the thumb.
• Swing the pinched index finger and the thumb from under the loop to the opposite side of the loop.
• Throw the active strand over the loop and grasp it between the pinched index finger and thumb.
• Pass the active strand through from under the loop.
• Grasp the active strand from under the loop and do not pull down.

b) After the completion of the first loop around the index finger, make a second loop again around the index finger (Figures 3.33 - 3.35) and only then pull the knot down (Figure 3.36).

c) Repeat all steps of unit two to complete the friction knot (Figure 3.37 - 3.40).

• Move the left thumb inside the passive strand and form a loop around the thumb using the active strand.
• Pinch the thumb and the index finger together.
• Swing the pinched thumb and index finger from under the loop to the opposite side and grasp the active strand.
• Pass the active strand through the loop.
• Grasp the active strand from under the loop and put the knot down with the help of index finger.

notes...

For all diagrams, the active strand is red and the passive strand is **black**.

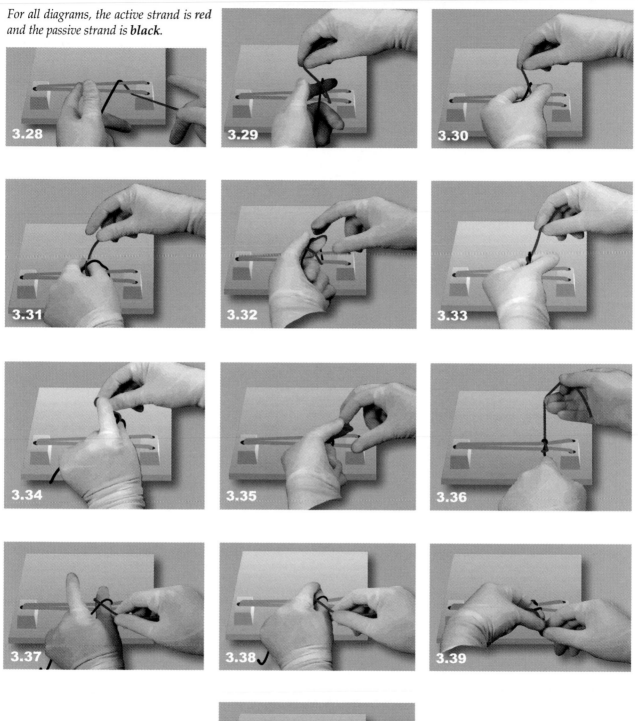

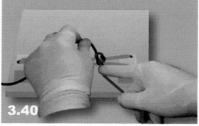

3:2:4 Sliding Knot

Sliding knots are used when the tension is extremely high for approximation of the wound (e.g. approximation of the ribs after a thoracotomy).

Steps:

a) Complete the first unit of a one-handed technique (Figure 3.41-3.45).

• For this knot, grasp the strands or segments of the suture with thumb and index finger and leave the three fingers, namely middle, ring and little fingers free for manipulation.
• Make a loop around the three fingers by moving the passive (black) strand over the top.
• Flex the middle finger to pull the active strand and grasp between the middle and ring fingers.
• Sweep the active strand from under the loop holding the active strand between the middle and ring fingers.
• Pull the knot slightly with the left index finger, but do not tie it down.

b) Repeat the same unit again and avoid overlapping the two knots (Figure 3.46 - 3.49).

c) Pull only one (passive black) strand toward oneself (Figure 3.50).

d) When the wound is approximated to satisfaction, pull the second (active red) strand in the opposite direction to lock the knot (Figure 3.51).

e) Complete the alternate unit of a one-handed technique to square and secure the knot (Figure 3.52 - 3.55).

• Grasp the active (red) strand with thumb and middle finger.
• Make a loop around the index finger by moving the index finger under the active (red) strand and bringing the passive (black) over the top of the index finger.
• Flex the left index finger catching the active (red) strand with the dorsum of the finger (fingernail).
• Sweep the active strand through the loop with the help of the index finger.
• Grasp the active strand from under the loop with the same hand and tighten with the index finger.

notes...

*For all diagrams, the active strand is red and the passive strand is **black**.*

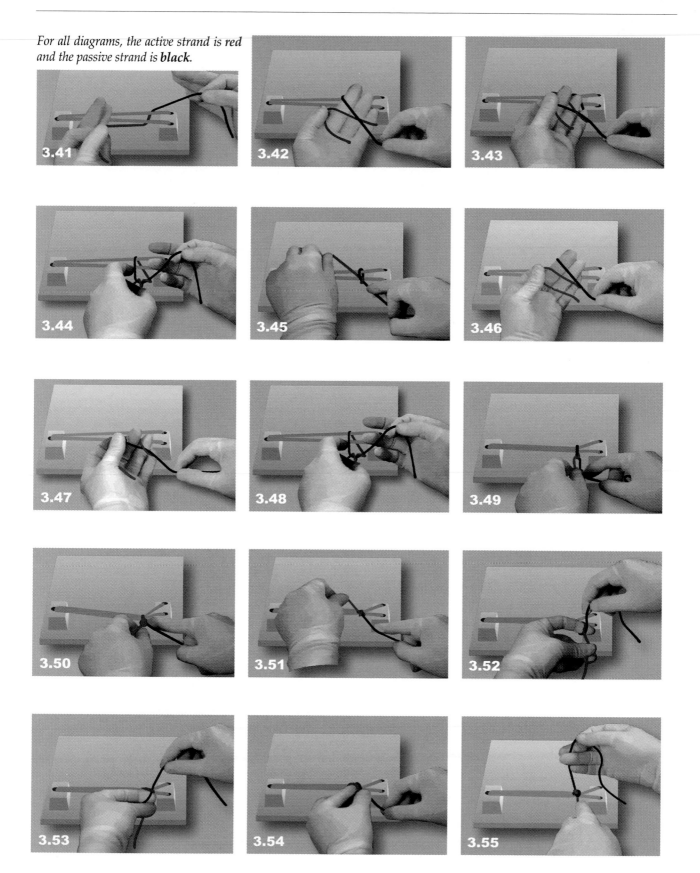

3:2:5 Instrument Tie

This technique is useful for the economy of suture materials or when a surgeon is working alone. This technique should be used only for superficial wounds.

a) Hold needle holder parallel with incision (Figure 3.56).

b) Form a loop around the instrument with the active (red) strand and grasp the end of the passive (black) strand (Figure 3.57).

c) Pull the passive strand under the loop (Figure 3.58).

d) Repeat the maneuvers described and form a loop in the opposite direction to form a square knot (Figures 3.59 - 3.61).

notes...

For all diagrams, the active strand is red
and the passive strand is **black***.*

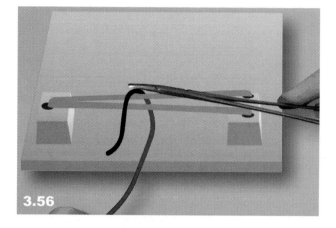

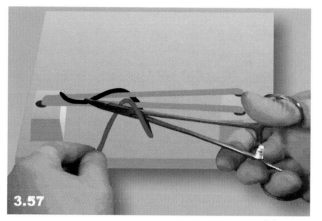

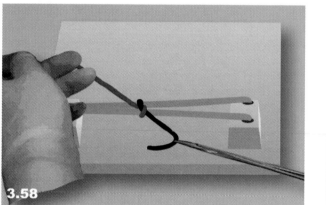

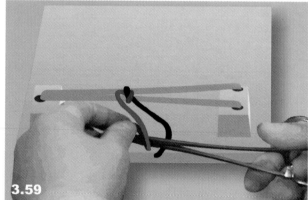

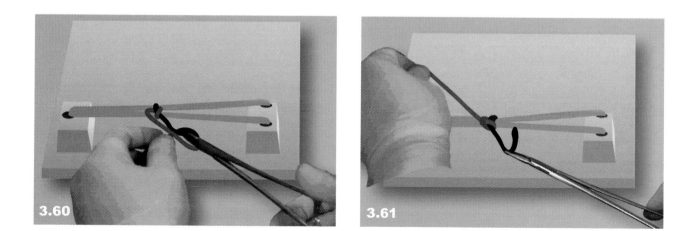

3:2:6 Friction Knot with Instrument Tie

a) Hold needle holder parallel with incision (Figure 3.62).

b) For this technique, make a double loop around the instrument with the active (red) strand and grasp the end of the passive strand (Figures 3.63 - 3.64).

c) Pull the passive strand under the loop (Figure 3.65).

d) Repeat the maneuvers described and form a loop in the opposite direction to make a square knot (Figures 3.66 - 3.68).

notes...

*For all diagrams, the active strand is red and the passive strand is **black**.*

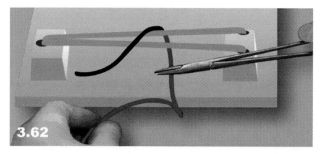

3.62

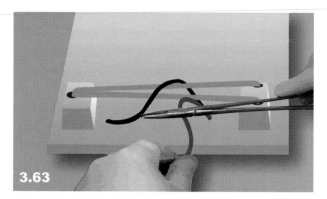

3.63

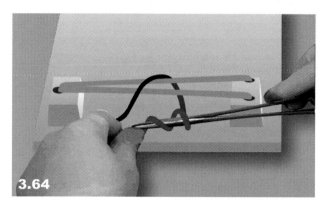

3.64

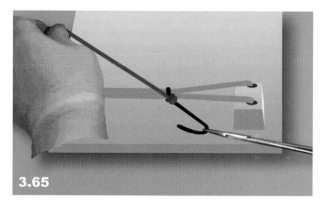

3.65

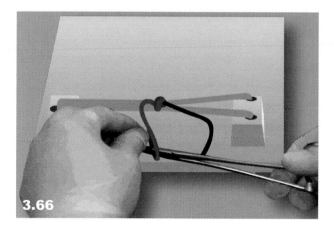

3.66

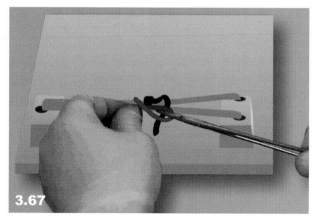

3.67

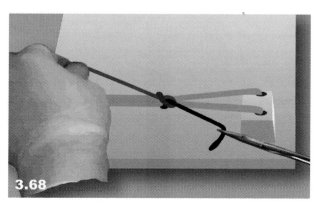

3.68

Chapter 4

Wound Management Techniques

Chapter 4		Contents	Page

Management of surgical wounds requires an intimate knowledge of wound healing and the factors which affect the healing process, local anesthetics and surgical techniques. This chapter will discuss only surgical principles and techniques used for wound management, including local anesthesia, hemostasis, tissue dissection, debridement, sewing and repair, as well as cutting and removing sutures.

4:1 Local Anesthesia

Local anesthesia is performed with anesthetic solutions such as xylocaine, lidocaine, marcaine and others. There are three basic techniques for local anesthesia: infiltration, field block, and nerve block.

4:1:1 Infiltration

In this technique, 0.5 - 1% xylocaine is injected throughout the area where the operation is planned. A 25 gauge needle (1/2 inch) is used first to raise a skin wheal (Figure 4.1). The underlying layers of tissue are then infiltrated with the use of a larger, longer needle (22 gauge, 1-1/2 inch).

4:1:2 Field Block

With this type of anesthesia, the field of surgery is blocked by infiltration of xylocaine (0.5-1%) around the area of operation (Figure 4.2). This technique is not used frequently.

4:1:3 Nerve Block

A nerve block includes the infiltration of local anesthesia around the nerve, in order to provide anesthesia in the distribution of that nerve, e.g. digital nerve block to repair finger lacerations (Figure 4.3). Intercostal nerve block is used for the management of pain due to chest trauma, intercostal neu-

ralgia or for post-operative pain management after thoracic surgery (Figure 4.4).

Nerve blocks can be performed with higher concentrations of xylocaine (1-2%) or marcaine (2%).

Technique for performance of a nerve block:

a) Formation of skin wheal with 25 gauge needle.

b) Insertion of a longer needle through the wheal to the targeted nerve. When the needle reaches the nerve, the patient feels paresthesia along the nerve distribution. At this point, the needle is withdrawn 2-3 mm.

c) Aspirate the needle to make sure that the needle is not in a blood vessel.

d) Inject 2-5 ml of 1-2% solution in the area surrounding the nerve.

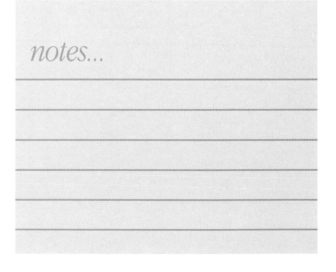

notes...

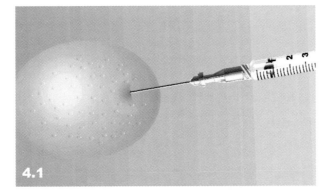

4.1

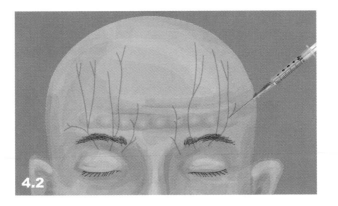

4.2

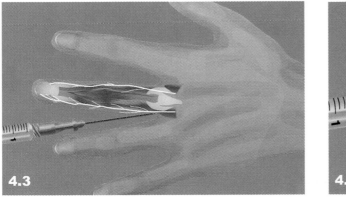

4.3

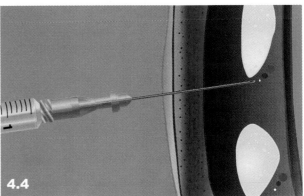

4.4

4:2 Hemostasis

This is the process of stopping or preventing the flow of blood from incised, transected or otherwise traumatized blood vessels.

Hemostasis techniques can be subdivided into the following major categories:

1) Temporary Hemostasis
2) Permanent Hemostasis

4:2:1 Temporary Methods of Hemostasis

Temporary methods of hemostasis include interruption of blood flow from the bleeding point by temporary measures. The following are basic techniques commonly used for this purpose:

a) Digital pressure on the bleeding point (Figure 4.5 - 4.6).

b) Pressing the supplying vessel proximally (for arteries) or distally (for veins) to the bleeding point (Figure 4.7).

c) Pressing the major arteries to the bone proximal to the bleeding area using pressure points: axilla, antecubital space, wrist, groin, and popliteal space. The carotid artery can be pressed to the processus transversus of C4 vertebrae (Figure 4.8).

d) Elevating the extremity upwards (Figure 4.9).

e) Applying a tourniquet (Figure 4.10).

NB: A tourniquet should be applied tightly and should not be kept on more than two hours. The tourniquet should be released every 20 minutes, for 1-2 minutes, and then re-applied.

f) Applying a clamp or forceps onto the artery (Figure 4.11).

g) Applying a biological, chemical or physical tamponade (Figure 4.12).

notes...

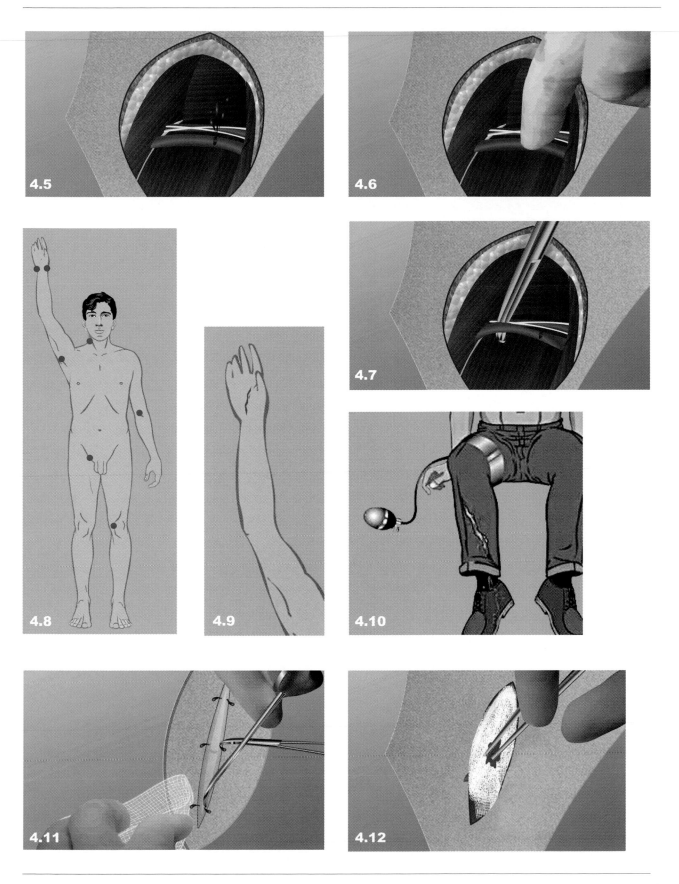

4.5

4.6

4.7

4.8

4.9

4.10

4.11

4.12

4:2:2 Permanent Methods of Hemostasis

Permanent methods of hemostasis include interruption of blood flow from the bleeding point by permanent measures.

The following are basic techniques commonly used for permanent hemostasis:

a) Ligation of the artery (Figure 4.13).

b) Tying the artery with the surrounding tissue into a figure 8 (Figure 4.14 - 4.15).

c) Sewing the lacerated or cut artery (Figure 4.16).

d) Application of biological or synthetic hemostatic material such as Surgicel, Gelfoam, pledgets or a piece of fat in order to seal a small laceration that may occur at the needle point in areas with soft tissue and high pressure (Figure 4.17).

e) Electro-coagulation of the bleeding points with a cautery (Figure 4.18).

f) Clipping. Permanent hemostasis can also be achieved with application of clips. The proximal side of the artery is clipped twice and the distal part requires one clip. Clips should be applied on a dissected and well-exposed artery. When the proximal and distal ends of the artery are clipped, only then can it be transected between the clips. (Figure 4.19).

Hemostasis can also be classified by factors which are utilized to stop bleeding:

a) Physical. Use of physical factors such as digital pressure applied to the bleeding points or proximal to the bleeding points are frequently used for hemostasis. The Pringle maneuver is a classic example of applying pressure proximal to the bleeding point (hepatic artery and portal vein in the hepatoduodenal ligament are clamped with non-crushing hemostatic forceps to control bleeding from the liver). Also used are a tourniquet application, and a bandage with pressure.

b) Temperature. Vasoconstriction by cooled temperatures and coagulation of bleeding vessels by high temperatures are classic examples for the use of temperature as a factor in hemostasis.

c) Chemical Agents. Use of vasoconstrictive agents and local hemostatic pads such as Surgicel are examples of chemical hemostasis.

d) Biological Agents. Materials such as platelets, fresh frozen plasma, and autogenous tissue are often used for hemostasis in surgery.

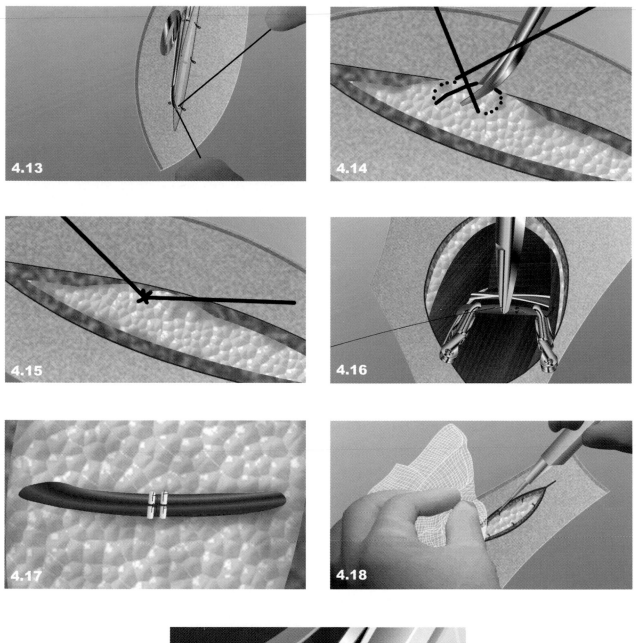

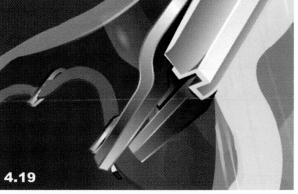

The most important technique of hemostasis, frequently used during surgical procedures, is the application of hemostatic clamps with subsequent ligation, suturing or coagulation of the blood vessel. The most commonly used hemostatic clamping techniques are as follows:

a) Hemostatic clamp applied at a bleeding point (Figure 4.20).

Steps for tying the bleeding point:

• The assistant holds the clamp upward at a 90° angle to the surgical plane, while the surgeon passes the suture from under the clamp and around the clamp (Figure 4.21).
• The assistant should show the end of the clamp to the surgeon by moving the clamp downward (parallel to the surgical plane) and to the side.
• Tie down with a simple knot (Figure 4.22).
• When the first knot is tightly in place, the clamp can be removed slowly while further tightening the knot (Figure 4.23).
• Apply subsequent knots and make sure that the knots are squared and are not less than three.

b) Hemostatic clamp applied before cutting the blood vessel.

Sometimes the knowledge of anatomy or visual observation of blood vessels give the surgeon a chance to prevent bleeding by applying clamps before cutting the vessel.

This technique includes the following steps:

• Isolate and dissect the tissue around the blood vessel and clamp the vessel proximally and distally (Figure 4.24).
• Cut the blood vessel (Figure 4.25).
• Tie the vessel with a ligature as described above.

notes...

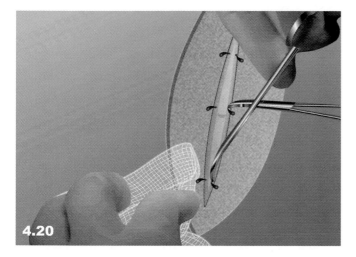

4.20

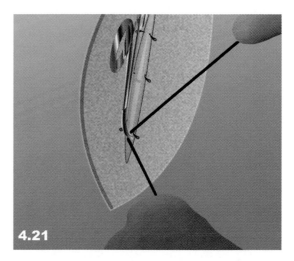

4.21

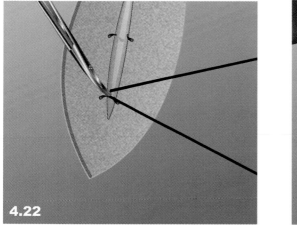

4.22

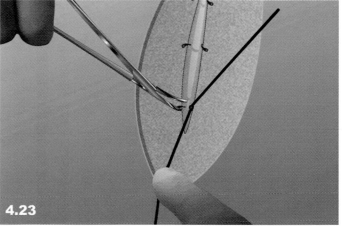

4.23

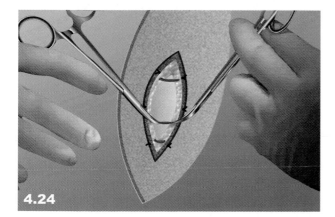

4.24

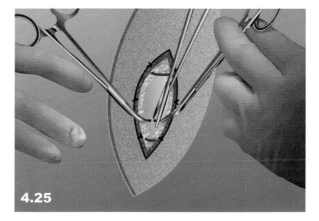

4.25

c) Sometimes the tissue is too thick or the end point of the clamp is not visible. In this case, the blood vessel can be sewn as follows:

• Place a suture under and close to the end of the clamp.
• Tie the end with a simple knot without taking the clamp out (Figure 4.26).
• Pass the tie from under the clamp (Figure 4.27).
• Tie down the entire tissue with slow removal of the clamp (Figure 4.28).

d) Sometimes it is difficult to control the bleeding point with a clamp because the elastic properties of cut arteries shorten, causing them to disappear in the tissue. Once the clamp is applied it is impossible for the operator to bring the tie around the blood vessel. In this case, a technique called "figure 8" suture ligation is used (Figure 4.29 - 4.31).

e) Applying two hemostatic clamps to a blood vessel before dividing may be traumatic and cause bleeding, especially from small fragile blood vessels. "Tying in continuity" consists of passing two ties under the dissected vessel and tying prior to cutting. This is the least traumatic method of hemostasis (Figure 4.32).

NB: Important rules for hemostasis:

• Do not panic.
• Use a temporary method to stop bleeding, i.e. applying pressure with fingers or gauze.
• A hard hemostat must not be applied blindly as it can cause more damage. Remember that every artery is accompanied by veins and nerves. Crushing the artery, vein or nerve is not a solution.
• Request appropriate soft clamps and other instruments.
• Expose the blood vessel proximally and distally.
• Apply the soft clamps and repair the blood vessel.
• If the situation becomes difficult, apply an appropriate temporary method and ask for help.

notes...

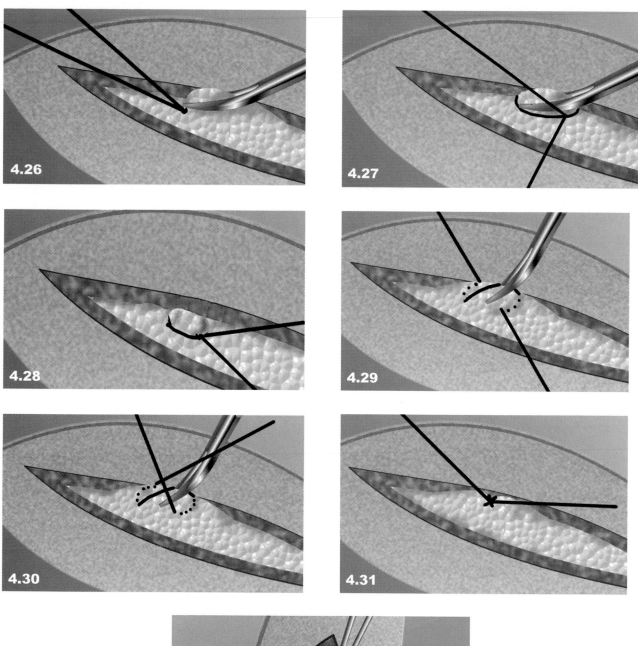

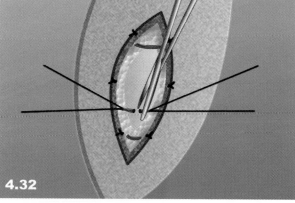

4:3 Tissue Dissection Techniques

Cutting, slicing, separating and isolating the tissue is called dissection. Tissue dissection techniques are used by surgeons to separate tissue planes or layers, and to isolate target structures for surgical manipulation. These techniques help reach organs, tissue structures such as tumors, anatomical landmarks and foreign bodies located in the depths of the tissue. These techniques are used consistently by surgeons in many operations.

Tissue dissection techniques can be subdivided into the following main categories:

4:3:1 Sharp Dissection

Tissue or certain planes can be cut simply with a sharp instrument. Sharp dissection is performed mainly with a scalpel (Figure 4.33) or scissors (Figure 4.34).

4:3:2 Blunt Dissection

Separation of tissue or layers and planes of tissue by pressure without cutting is called blunt dissection. Blunt dissection can be performed with instruments such as scissors or by the fingers (Figure 4.35).

4:3:3 Combined Sharp and Blunt Dissection

Combined sharp and blunt dissection can also be performed with sharp instruments by cutting while pushing the instrument toward the desired direction (Figure 4.36-4.37).

All these techniques can be performed with an electrocautery. In extensive surgical procedures, dissection with electrocautery is preferred due to the capacity of the instrument to cut and coagulate at the same time. This facilitates dissection with simultaneous hemostasis.

Undermining is a dissection technique used mostly for approximation of skin defects. The tissue is dissected under the skin flap in order to make the skin more flexible for approximation (Figure 4.38).

Another useful technique is the use of instruments, such as scissors or a clamp, under the target tissue aimed for cutting so that the target tissue can be elevated in order to protect the underlying vital tissue from unnecessary trauma (Figure 4.39).

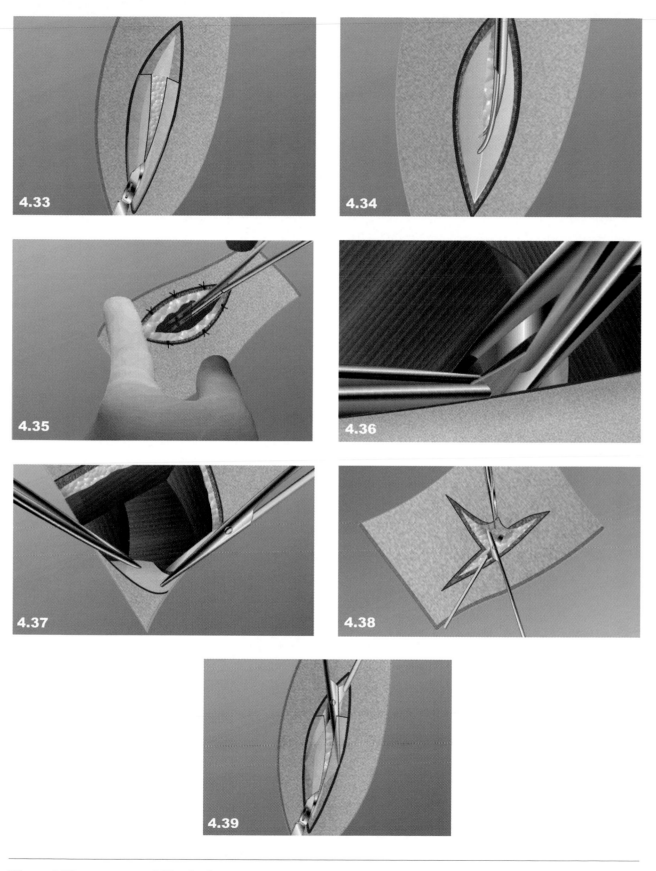

4:4 Basic Technique for Wound Repair

Wound closure is subdivided into three categories:

4:4:1 Closure by Primary Intent

The wound is closed in 8-12 hours for extremities and 24 hours for facial lacerations

4:4:2 Closure by Secondary Intent

The wound is not closed and allowed to granulate on its own without surgical closure

4:4:3 Closure by Tertiary Intent (also called Delayed Primary Closure)

The wound is initially left open to granulate, and then is sutured, usually 3-4 days later.

4:5 Debridement

Debridement is a technique used for repair of laceration and non-sterile wounds.

Steps:

a) infiltration of local anesthesia (for small wounds) (Figure 4.40).

b) washing the wound with saline for mechanical cleaning of dirt, debris or other foreign bodies (Figure 4.41).

c) if this is not sufficient, about 1 mm of the wound edge should be trimmed (Figure 4.42).

d) ensure the excision evens the edges of the wound (Figure 4.43).

e) ensure all the necrotic or severely damaged tissue is removed.

f) the clean (free of foreign bodies and necrotic tissue), even edges of the wound are sewn together (Figure 4.44 - 4.45).

notes...

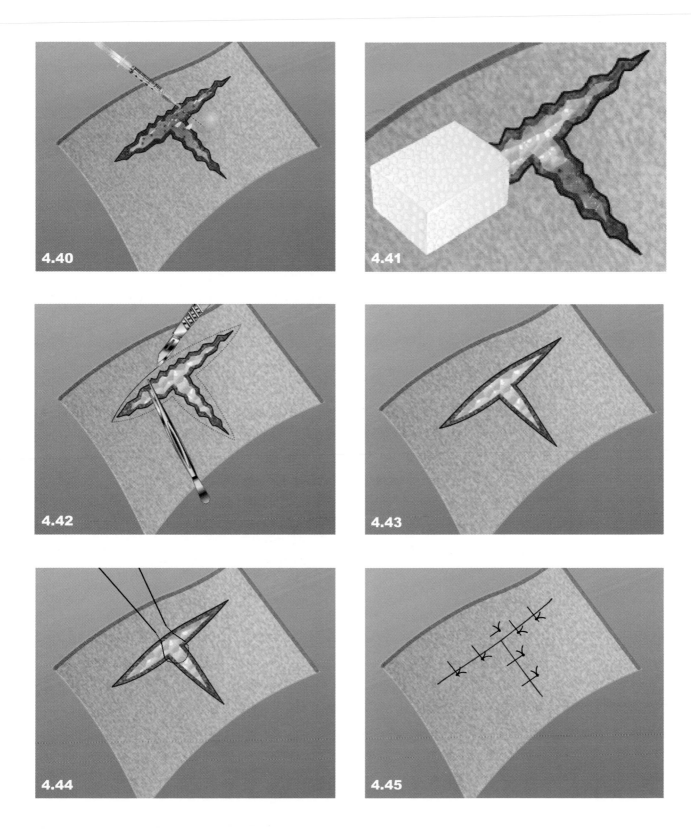

4.40

4.41

4.42

4.43

4.44

4.45

4:6 Principles of Sewing and Repair

a) the wound should be approximated to eliminate any dead space or empty pockets (Figures 4.46 - 4.47).

b) the edges of the wound should be everted, not inverted or overlapped (Figures 4.48 - 4.50).

c) it may be necessary to extend the end of the wound to make the wound more flexible.

d) in a case where the edges of the wound are difficult to bring together and the maneuver creates a great deal of tension, use the undermining technique (see pp. 80 - 81).

NB: Skin tension lines must be taken into consideration. This is found by pressing the skin in the area between the index finger and the thumb, or movement of the skin in the area of concern (Figure 4.51).

notes...

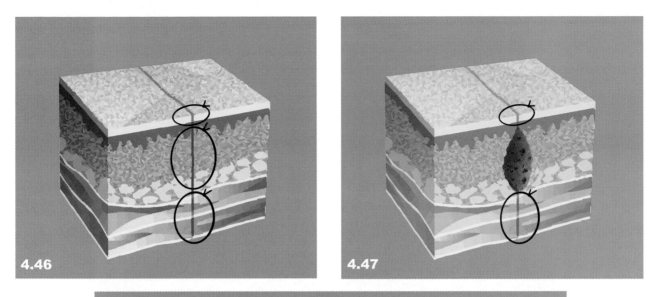

4.46

4.47

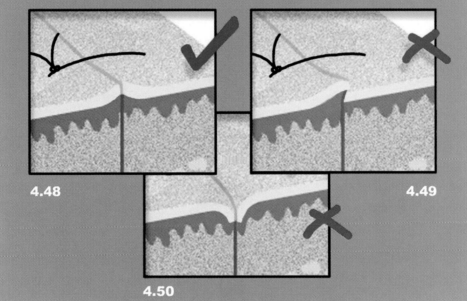

4.48

4.49

4.50

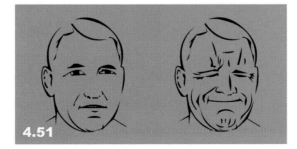

4.51

4:7 Wound Suturing Techniques

In this section, only the basic skin closure techniques are described. Special suturing techniques are discussed elsewhere. Basically, suturing techniques are divided into interrupted and continuous sutures.

4:7:1 Interrupted Sutures

With this technique, each suture is independent; that is, tied separately after the completion of each individual suture. The most commonly used interrupted sutures are:

a) Simple Interrupted Suture (Figure 4.52 - 4.54). This is the most commonly used interrupted suture. With this technique, equal bites of tissue should be taken on each side of the wound. The distance between the edge of the wound and the needle puncture can vary depending on the thickness of skin, however, a distance of 0.5 cm from the edge of the wound and between the sutures is usually sufficient to properly close the wound. Several layers of interrupted sutures may be required for proper repair, depending on the depth of the wound. For example, for repair of a wound that has reached the muscles, the first suture layer is placed in the muscle sheath, the second in the superficial fascia and the third in the skin. The advantage of interrupted sutures is that in the case of loosening or removal of one suture, the integrity of the wound is held by other sutures; for example, in the case of wound infection, by removing one suture, it is possible to drain the pus and keep the rest of the wound together.

NB: It is very important for the edges of the wound to be everted after interrupted sutures are completed. If this is not achieved during suturing and tying, the edges can be everted using two pick-up forceps after the wound is closed.

notes...

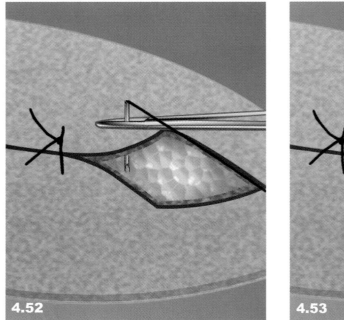

4.52

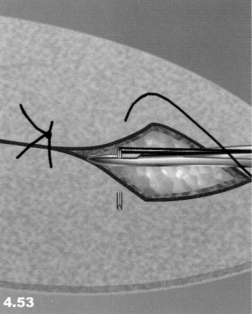

4.53

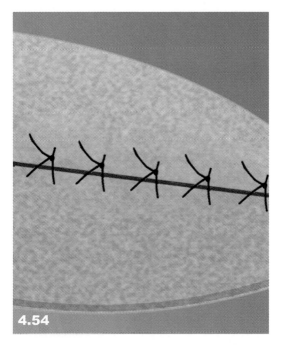

4.54

b) Vertical Mattress Suture. Vertical mattress suture takes both deep and superficial bites in one suture.

• The first bite of this suture enters the skin further away from the edge of the wound than the simple interrupted suture (about 1.0 cm), and reaches under the superficial fascia inside the wound (Figure 4.55).

• The suture then comes out with the same distance and depth through the near side of the wound (Figure 4.56).

• The second bites are back-handed and pass only through the most superficial cuticular or subcuticular layers of dermis on both sides of the wound (Figure 4.57).

• Figure 4.58 demonstrates the completion of the vertical mattress suture. The advantage of this suture is that it covers deep wounds without leaving a "dead" space that facilitates the accumulation of fluid and predisposes the wound to infection. This suture also everts the edges of the wound providing the most optimal healing conditions for the skin.

notes...

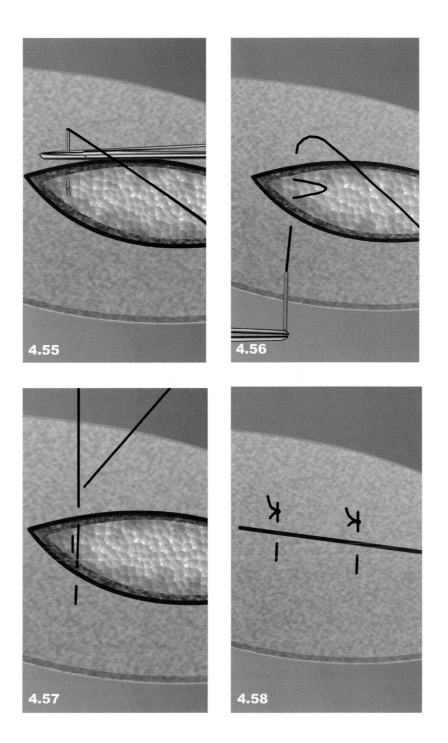

4.55

4.56

4.57

4.58

c) Horizontal Mattress Suture. Both bites of this suture are placed horizontally, i.e. parallel to the wound edges (Figures 4.59 - 4.61).

d) Inverted Interrupted Suture. In this technique, the needle enters beneath the target layer and comes out from the top on the near side of the wound (deep to superficial). On the far side, the needle enters from the top of the target layer and comes out beneath the target layer (superficial to deep). When the suture is tied, the knots skip under the suture and they cannot been seen on the surface of the wound (i.e. the knots are buried) (Figures 4.62 - 4.64). This technique is used mostly in subcutaneous closure or initiation of a continuous suture. It is also used in closure of superficial layers such as the platysma muscle in the neck. Since large knots would be visible under the skin, this method is cosmetically unacceptable.

notes...

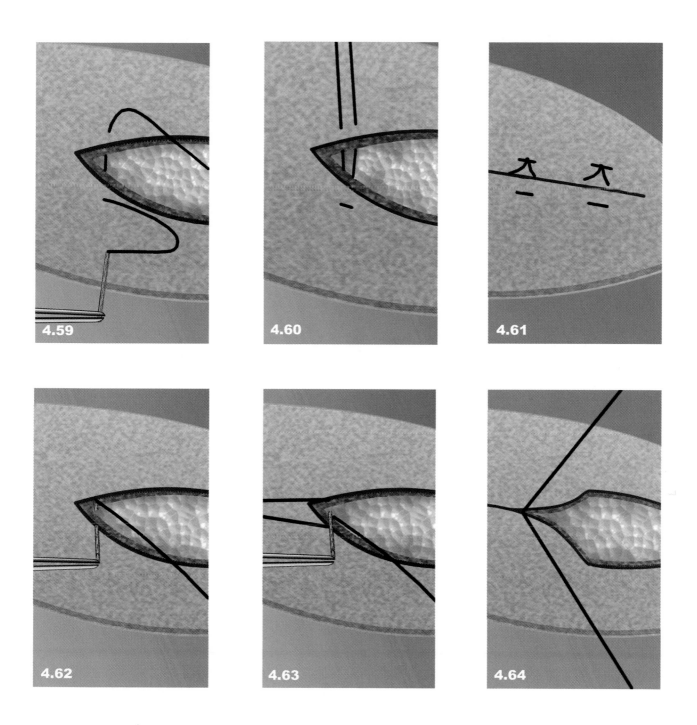

4.59

4.60

4.61

4.62

4.63

4.64

e) Semi-Mattress Suture. Semi-mattress sutures are an excellent technique used for laceration repair and/or uneven wounds with a variety of geometric forms and configurations.

• The first bite of this suture enters the skin further away from the edge of the wound as in the vertical mattress or horizontal mattress suture (Figure 4.65).

• On the near side of the wound, the suture does not go through the skin. It grabs only the subcuticular layer of the skin (Figure 4.66).

• The next bite is back-handed and passes through the dermis most superficially only on the far side of the wound (Figure 4.67). It can also come out beside the first suture as in the horizontal mattress suture.

notes...

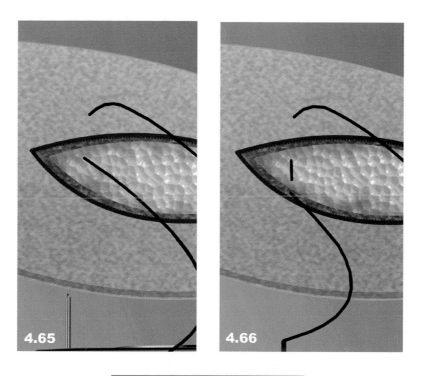

4.65

4.66

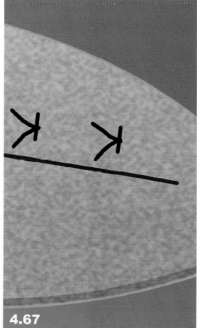

4.67

4:7:2 Continuous Sutures

In this technique, approximation of the edges of the wound is achieved by continuous placement of sutures without tying and cutting the suture material. Continuous sutures have certain advantages over interrupted sutures:

a) can be completed faster and therefore have a time-saving effect.

b) are able to adjust and accommodate postoperative edema of the wound edges.

The major disadvantage is that the integrity of the wound is in jeopardy if one of the sutures is cut off.

Continuous sutures can be divided into:

a) Simple Continuous Suture (Figure 4.68 - 4.72). The suture starts from the far edge of the wound about 0.5 cm away from the edge, entering the wound from outside in, and exiting from inside out, on the near edge of the wound. After the suture is tied, it can be continued on with the needle pathway of a 45° or a 90° angle to the wound. To end this suture, the last passage should be made about 3 mm from the corner of the wound. The needle is then passed from the same side about 2 mm apart from the last exit to the far side of the wound. The suture is then tied down with a loop left on the near side.

notes...

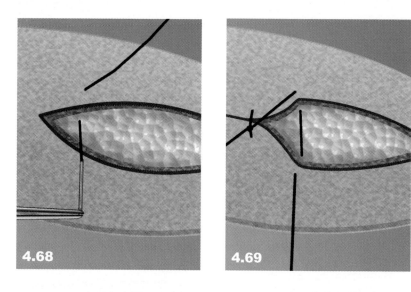

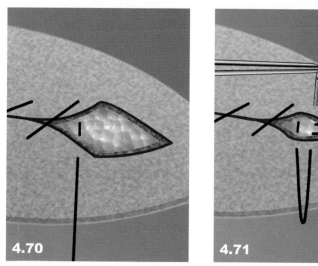

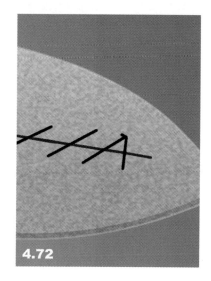

b) Interlocking Continuous Sutures. In this type of suture, the needle is passed through the loop made by the previous suture. The rest of the procedure is similar to the simple continuous suture using a needle placement of a 90° angle to the wound edges (Figure 4.73 - 4.75).

c) Horizontal Mattress Continuous Suture. This is also called continuous inverting mattress suture. This suture is similar to the interrupted horizontal mattress suture with a parallel arm to the edge of the wound. In order to accomplish this task, when the needle is passed from outside in, it should then be passed from inside out on the same side of the wound parallel to the port of entry (Figure 4.76 - 4.78).

notes...

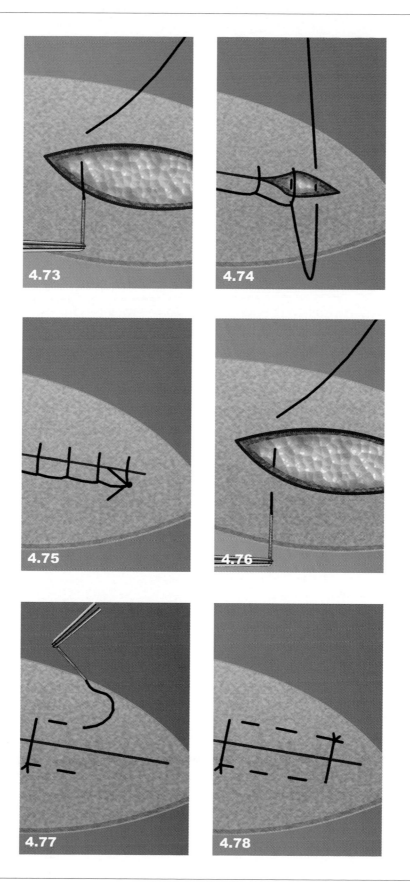

4.73

4.74

4.75

4.76

4.77

4.78

d) Subcuticular Suture. This suture gives good skin closure by approximating the subcuticular layers. It has the advantages of better cosmetic scar and better blood supplies for the healing process. The suture should be anchored at one end of the wound and then inserted into the subcuticular layers of the tissue parallel to the skin. The suture is not pulled tight until the full suture has been placed. After it has been pulled taut, the distal end is also anchored. Anchors can be outside or inside the wound. An absorbable suture with an inverted inside anchor is preferred (Figure 4.79 - 4.82).

Continuous sutures must not be used on wounds that are predisposed to infection. The disadvantage of this suture is that if it is broken in one place the entire wound will open.

NB: Do not use continuous sutures on the skin unless the wound is cut in sterile conditions and the possibility of infection from opening of the internal organ does not exist.

e) Stapling. The skin wound can also be closed with the use of staples. Staples are as efficient as sutures and they can be applied much faster. There are several stapling devices on the market, however, staplers with a rotating head provides better visualization of the wound. In addition to the speed of wound closure, it has been proven that use of staples reduces wound complications such as infection in comparison to reactive surgical sutures.

Technique:

• Place the stapler perpendicular to the length of the wound at a 90° angle to the skin (Figure 4.83).
• The arrow on the cartridge should point to the incision line where the tack is placed (inset, Figure 4.84).
• Press the stapler to the skin firmly.
• Squeeze the handle of the loading unit completely (Figure 4.84).
• Release the handle completely.
• Reposition the stapler and repeat the procedure.

notes...

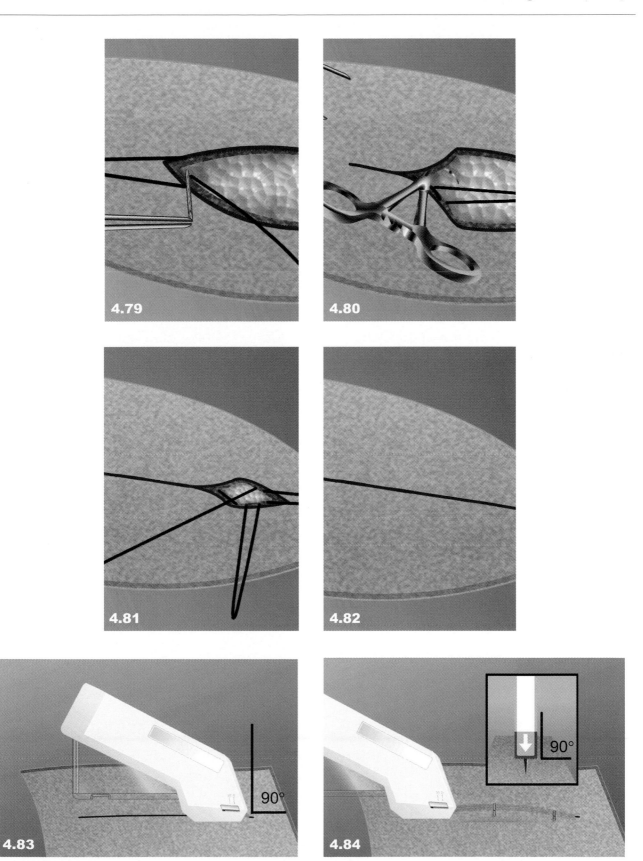

4.79

4.80

4.81

4.82

4.83

90°

4.84

90°

4:8 Cutting Sutures

Sutures should neither be cut very close to the knots nor far away from the knots. If they are cut too close to the knot, there is the possibility of them becoming untied; if they are cut too long, an additional, undesirable foreign body will be left in the wound. Silk sutures hold knots well (do not unravel) and should be cut about 1-2 mm above the knot. In order to achieve this objective, the tip of the scissors should be pushed down to the knot and then turned to the side (Figure 4.85 - 4.86). Some synthetic materials tend to unravel and it is better to cut 4-6 mm above the knot. On the other hand, skin sutures must be left with longer ends to facilitate suture removal (Figure 4.87 - 4.88).

4:9 Removing Sutures

Sutures can be removed in seven days for most parts of the body. However, in the face and neck they can be removed earlier (3-5 days). Retention sutures should be left longer (10-14 days).

Steps:

• Pick up the end of the suture above the knots with forceps (Figure 4.89).

• Pull the suture slightly up to be able to place the tip of the scissors under the suture (Figure 4.90).

• Divide the suture where it dips beneath the skin (Figure 4.91).

• Gently pull the suture out through the other skin orifice.

notes...

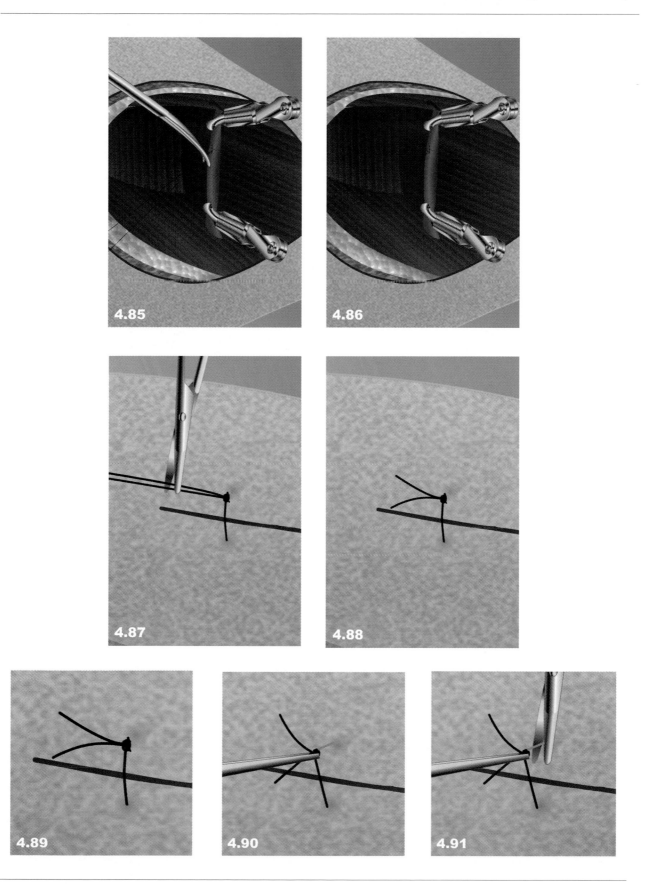

4.85

4.86

4.87

4.88

4.89

4.90

4.91

Chapter 5

Aseptic Techniques and Operating Room Conduct

Judith S. Fialkow, R.N. BScN, CPN(C)

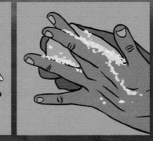

Chapter 5   *Contents*   *Page*

Up until the second half of the 19th Century, the vast majority of surgical operations were complicated with wound infection, mainly due to the lack of knowledge about microbes. In 1867, Louis Pasteur discovered micro-organisms and described the presence of these microscopic beings in the fermentation process. A year later, Joseph Lister described the presence of microorganisms in infected wounds and proved that microbes are, in fact, the etiological sources of infected surgical wounds. He subsequently described a method that can destroy the microbes in the wound, called antisepsis ("anti" from the Latin prefix against and "sepsis" infection).

Originally, Lister proposed 3% carbolic acid as an antiseptic (antiseptics are chemical agents used for destruction of micro-organisms). This antisepsis method soon became unpopular and caused frustration among surgeons mainly due to two reasons:

a) Antiseptics such as 3% carbolic acid destroyed tissue as well as microbes in the wound causing necrosis, and at times, more problems for the surgeon.

b) Some microbes became adapted to the carbolic acid and hence the antiseptic solution was no longer useful for destruction of micro-organisms in the wound.

In the midst of these difficulties, a young surgeon and investigator, Semmelweis, came up with a new idea. He proposed destruction of the microbes before they came into contact with surgical wounds. This method was called asepsis ("*a*" - from Latin prefix *without* or *no* and "*sepsis*", infection). According to the principals of this method, every object including surgical instruments, surgeons' hands, clothing, drapes, sutures, and any other material that contacts the surgical wound, as well as the skin of the patient, is disinfected before surgery. The introduction of this method brought a great deal of success in the development of modern surgical treatment. Today, both aseptic and antiseptic techniques are used together for the successful performance of surgical operations. This chapter is a very brief introduction to, and an overview of, aseptic techniques and operating room conduct.

notes...

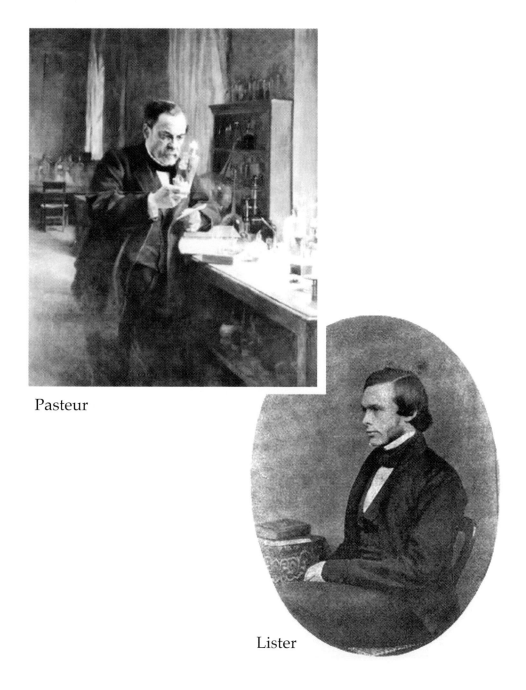

Pasteur

Lister

5:1 Principles of Aseptic Technique

The main objective of asepsis is to prevent the contamination of surgical wounds. For realization of this purpose, three important principals should be taken into consideration:

a) Prevention of contamination from air

b) Prevention of contamination from contact

c) Prevention of contamination from implantation

5:1:1 Prevention of Contamination from Air

Prevention of air contamination is accomplished by donning surgical masks, hats, shoes and special clothing before entering the restricted area, cleaning of the operating room with antiseptics, and 20-25 air exchanges, etc. Additional measures for prevention of air contamination include restriction of talking, moving and entry of additional personnel into the operating room (OR). In order to reduce the talking and noise in the OR, a type of sign language may be used. The following signs are widely accepted:

a) Asking for hemostatic clamp. Extend the hand supinely as shown in Figure 5.1. The palm must be open and upward, and the back of the hand toward the table.
b) Asking for scissors. Extend the index and middle fingers and separate them like the branches of scissors while flexing the other fingers (Figure 5.2).
c) Asking for scalpel. Extend the hand and keep thumb, index and middle fingers together as in holding a pencil (Figure 5.3).
d) Asking for forceps. Extend the thumb and index finger parallel to each other while flexing the other three fingers (Figure 5.4).
e) Asking for needle holder with a suture. Extend the hand with flexed finger as shown in Figure 5.5 with a motion from a pronation to supination.
f) Asking for a tie. Extend hand with extended fingers in a way that the back of the hand is toward the scrub nurse (Figure 5.6).

notes...

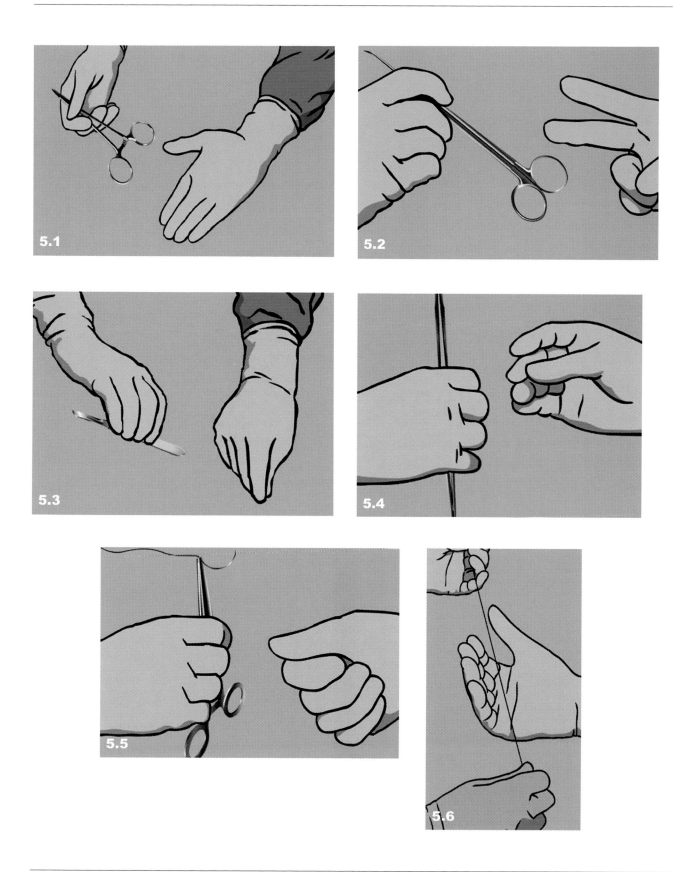

5:1:2 Prevention of Contamination from Contact

For prevention of contact contamination everything that comes in contact with, or that will surround the operating field, should be free of micro-organisms (sterile). Sterilization is a process which frees the material from bacteria, viruses, spores, and other micro-organisms. Surgeons, surgical assistants and nurses who are in direct contact with a surgical wound should scrub hands, don sterile gloves and proper sterile gowns, before approaching the operating field and wound contact. It is also extremely important to protect oneself from contamination by the patient.

The following specific measures are taken for prevention of infection caused by contact contamination from medical staff to patient, or vice versa:

5:1:2:1 Sterilization of Surgical Materials

There are various methods used to sterilize equipment, instrumentation and surgical supplies. The choice of method depends on the nature of the item to be sterilized.

The three methods are:

a) Thermal

i) Steam under pressure. An autoclave is widely used for metal instrumentation (Figure 5.7 - 5.8)

ii) Hot air/Dry heat
iii) Non-ionizing radiation/microwave

b) Chemical

i) Ethylene oxide (commonly used with items that are sensitive to heat).
ii) Formaldehyde gas
iii) Hydrogen peroxide plasma/vapor
iv) Ozone gas
v) Glutaraldehyde activated solution
vi) Peracetic Acid solution

c) Ionizing radiation

i) Radiation (physical)
ii) Gamma radiation

There are several indicators for monitoring the sterilization process.

a) Mechanical Indicators

• Sterilizers have gauges, thermometers, recorders and timers to monitor their function.

b) Chemical Indicators

• These are placed inside or outside of a package and verify exposure to a sterilization process. i.e. tape, paper strips etc. (Figure 5.9). If the tape does not have the desired result after sterilization (colour change) then it should not be used (Figure 5.10).

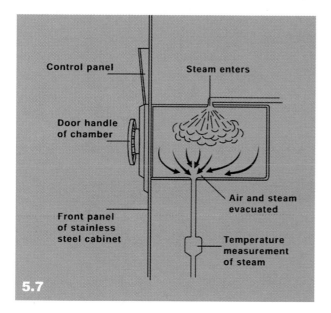

Control panel

Steam enters

Door handle
of chamber

Air and steam
evacuated

Front panel
of stainless
steel cabinet

Temperature
measurement
of steam

5.7

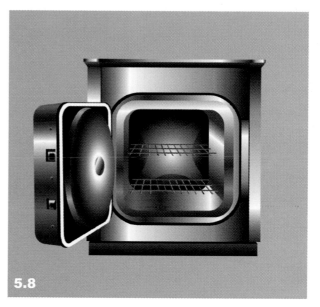

5.8

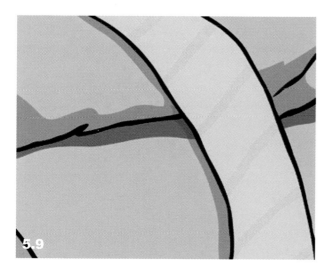

5.9

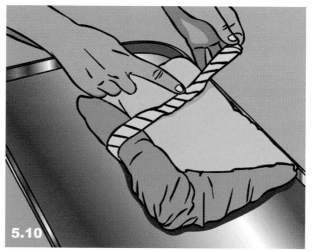

5.10

c) Biological Indicators

• These are usually live spores contained in small vials which are destroyed during sterilization.

5:1:2:2 Maintaining Integrity of Sterilized Items

All sterile items should be kept on a dry, clean, covered shelf. Care should be taken not to over-crowd or bend these items. If an item (cloth or paper wrapped) falls on the floor it should be considered unsterile due to "strike through" (microorganisms entering the package on impact). If materials become wet they are also considered unsterile due to microorganisms entering via the moist pathway.

NB: There is no compromise when it comes to sterility.

Before opening a sterile package it must be inspected for:

a) sterile indicator
b) absence of holes
c) integrity of seal

Opening a sterile item:

a) Package

• open away from oneself first (Figure 5.11)
• open side flaps next
• towards oneself last
• hold back all unsterile portions when presenting to the scrubbed person (Figure 5.12)

b) Peel Back Wrapper

• the peel should be pulled back to expose the sterile item

5:1:2:3 Body Substance Precautions

Every patient is considered a potentially contaminated source when blood or body fluids are involved. Although great care is taken to protect patients from staff source of contaminations, (hair, skin, respiratory etc.), the staff in turn must protect themselves from blood/fluid born pathogens.

The following protective barriers are used:

a) Gloves, latex (Figure 5.13). Double gloving is recommended for procedures > 2 hrs. or when large amounts of blood are anticipated .

NB: Always wash hands after gloves are removed.

b) Masks. Are used for protection from aerosols or droplets (Figure 5.14).

c) Eyewear/Goggles or Face shield. Are used to protect against aerosols, splashes or droplets (Figure 5.15).

d) Gowns. Made of fluid resistant materials and used to protect from body substances.

NB: Special care must be taken with all sharps.

• Always pass a knife/scalpel handle first and indicate to the scrub nurse that a scalpel or sharp is being handed back.
• Always use an instrument to attach or remove a blade.
• When finished stitching, always place the needle back on the needle driver and hand back to the scrub nurse.
• Use one handed capping method or do not cap at all and place directly in a sharps container (Figure 5.16).

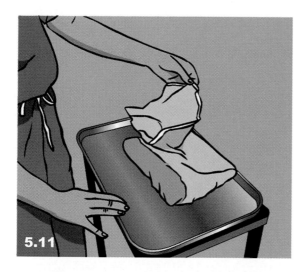

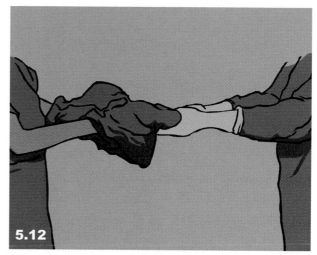

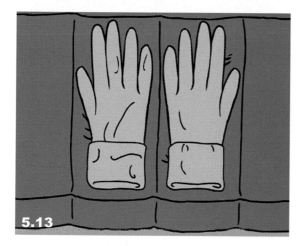

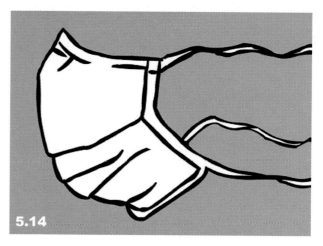

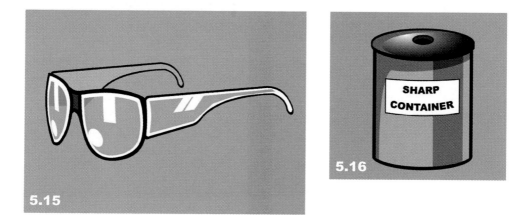

5:1:2:4 Scrubbing

Procedure:

• Before scrubbing, make sure a scrub cap is available. All of the hair must be completely covered. The mouth and nose must be comfortably covered with a mask (Figure 5.17).
• Wash both hands to about 2 inches above the elbows with soap and water.
• Take a scrub sponge and/or brush, open the package, wet the sponge and start scrubbing (Figure 5.18).
• Clean fingernails under running water (Figure 5.19).

NB:Remember that from now on nothing should be touched that is not sterile.

• The order of scrubbing starts from:
- the tip of the fingers (Figure 5.20)
- all sides of each finger (Figure 5.21)
- all planes of the hands (Figure 5.22)
- continue all planes up to the elbow (Figure 5.23)
• do not return to the hand once completed
• 5 minutes for 1st scrub of the day and 3 minutes for subsequent scrubs

Remember: hands first, then arms and elbows last for scrubbing and rinsing (Figure 5.24).

• When you are rinsing or scrubbing, the elbow should be bent upward so the water from the elbow does not go to the fingers and vice versa; the flow of water should be toward the elbow.

• To dry hands and arms, pick up a towel or wait until the towel is given to you. Keep hands and elbows away from body in an open space.
- with one side of the towel, dry fingers first (Figure 5.25)
- then the arm up to the elbow (Figure 5.26)
- flip the towel to the clean side (Figure 5.27)
- dry the other hand in the same fashion
- throw the towel into the laundry basket

NB: Do not take the towel from the nurses back table. The towel will be handed to you. If the gown and towel is set up on a separate small table then the towel may be taken by oneself. Be careful not to drip on the sterile field.

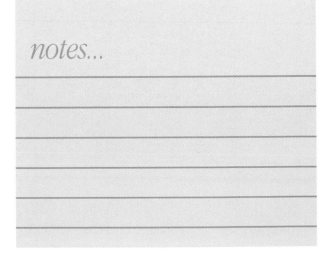

notes...

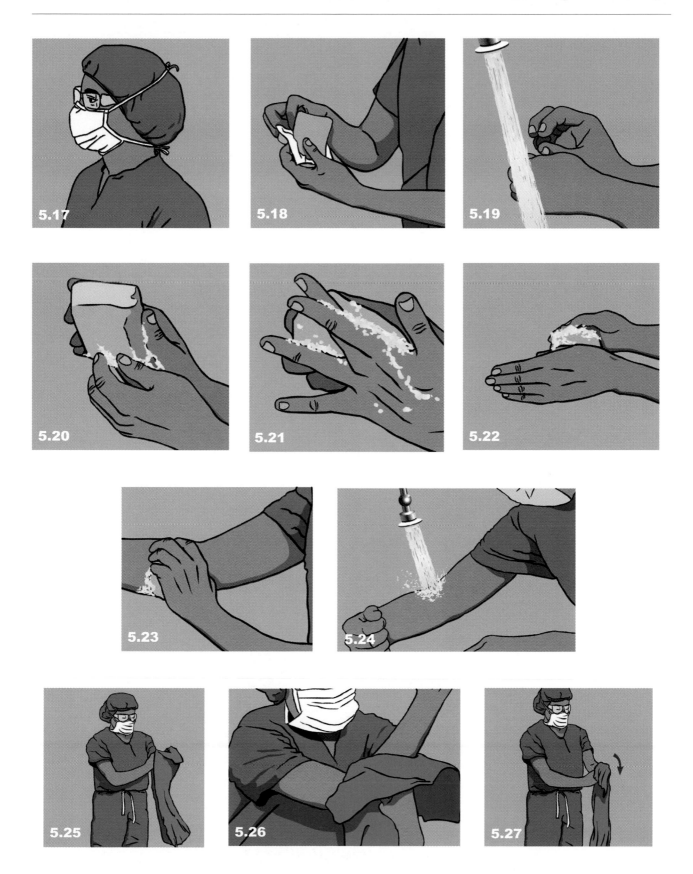

5:1:2:5 Gowning Yourself (closed technique)

The procedure for putting on a sterile gown when gowning oneself:

• Pick up the gown (from the small table) (Figure 5.28).
• Find an open space.
• Unfold the gown until the armholes are found.
• Place both hands into the armholes and advance them to the sleeves (Figure 5.29). Do not take hands out of the sleeves (Figure 5.30). Ensure that the sleeves do not flip back and touch unscrubbed upper arm. Protect sleeves as the arms enter (Figure 5.31).
• Ask for help (circulating nurse) to secure and adjust your gown (Figure 5.32 - 5.33).

NB: When gowning oneself the gown will be opened on a separate table. **Do not** gown off the main set up (scrub nurses table).

notes...

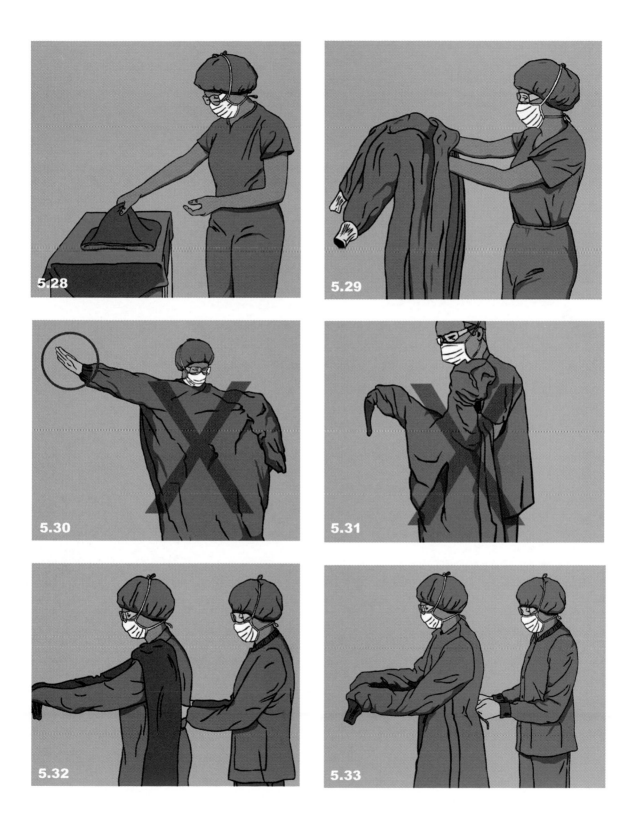

5:1:2:6 Gloving Yourself (closed technique)

The procedure for putting on sterile gloves when gloving oneself:

• Take the glove.
• Open it in a sterile environment (still having hands inside the sleeves).
• For "closed" technique of gloving, do not pull hands through the sleeve. Grasp the right glove in the left hand and turn the right hand so that the palm is upward.
• Place the right glove on the palm in such a way that the thumb of the glove is against the thumb (thumb to thumb) and the fingers of the glove are toward the body. In other words, flip the glove over so that the fingers are now toward the elbow (Figure 5.34).
• Bring thumb under the cuff of the glove, hook the glove with thumb and grasp securely (Figure 5.35).
• Flip the glove over fingers (Figure 5.36).
• Grab the glove and the sleeve together. Work fingers into the glove and pull the glove upward (Figure 5.37).

NB: Do not adjust the fingertips if fingers are not placed properly into the glove compartments.

• Repeat the same maneuvers for left hand (Figures 5.38 - 5.41)

NB: Only when both hands are in the gloves can the fingertips be adjusted (Figure 5.42).

If the gown is single tie, approach the sterile table.

If gown is double tie:

• Untie the bow knot.
• If another sterile person is not available, then a sterile clamp may be attached to the longest tie. The clamp is then passed to the unsterile person who will help you complete the turn.
• Turn your body around counterclockwise
• Grab the right end back and tie the ends (5.43 - 5.44).
• If there is another scrub (sterile) person, they may turn you. Hand the longer tie to the scrub person and turn around until the back of the gown is closed. Tie the ends together and let go. It is not permissable to touch these ends once they are dropped.

notes...

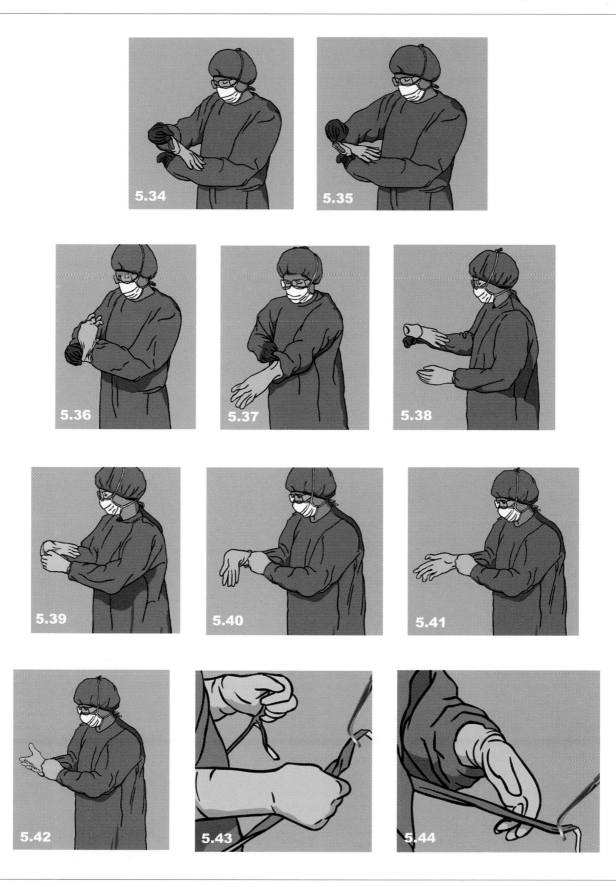

5:1:2:7 Gowned by the Scrub Nurse (open technique)

• After scrubbing and drying hands, the nurse will bring a gown fully expanded (Figure 5.45).

• Place hands into armholes (Figure 5.46)

• Gently advance hands into sleeves. At this time, the nurse leaves the gown on the shoulders therefore the hands must be kept upward to prevent the gown from falling down (Figure 5.47)

• The circulating nurse will grab the gown by placing a hand under the gown, thereby protecting his/her gloved hands, and grasping the gown from inside. When the nurse is pulling the gown over shoulders pull the sleeves over the hand. The circulating nurse is then able to tie the back ties.

• Figure 5.48 shows the improper position of the hand by the scrub nurse and Figure 5.49 demonstrates the proper position of the hand by the scrub nurse.

NB: This is an open technique and therefore the hands are allowed to be pulled from the sleeves.

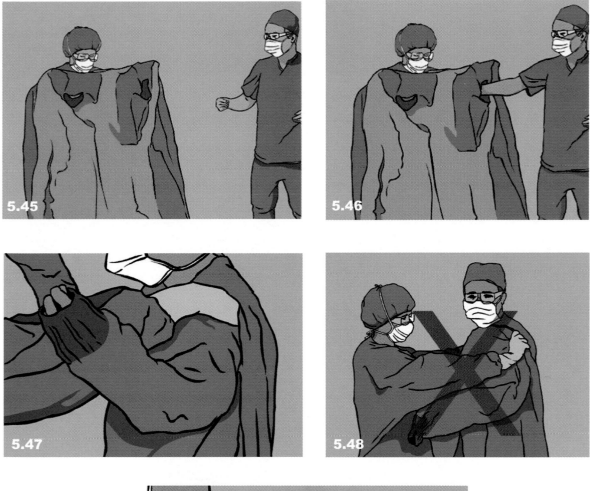

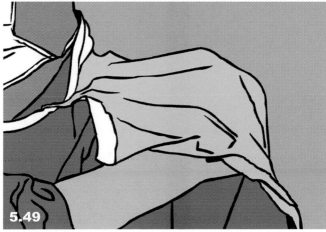

5:1:2:8 Gloving Done by the Scrub Nurse (open technique)

• The nurse opens the wrist portion of the glove (Figure 5.50).
• Place hand carefully into the glove compartment (Figure 5.51). Do not attempt to dive too low.
• Once the fingers are in the finger holes of the glove, slide hand further and the nurse at this time pulls the glove up
• For the left hand, it is advisable to help the nurse by pulling out the nearest cuff portion with the gloved hand.

NB: Only when both gloves are done may the fingers be adjusted (Figures 5.52 -5.53).

Note: Some surgical procedures pose a greater risk of the possibility of a glove puncture (e.g. orthopedics, where sharp reamers are commonly handled). In these instances it is highly recommended to double glove. It is policy in some hospitals to routinely double glove as added protection.

notes...

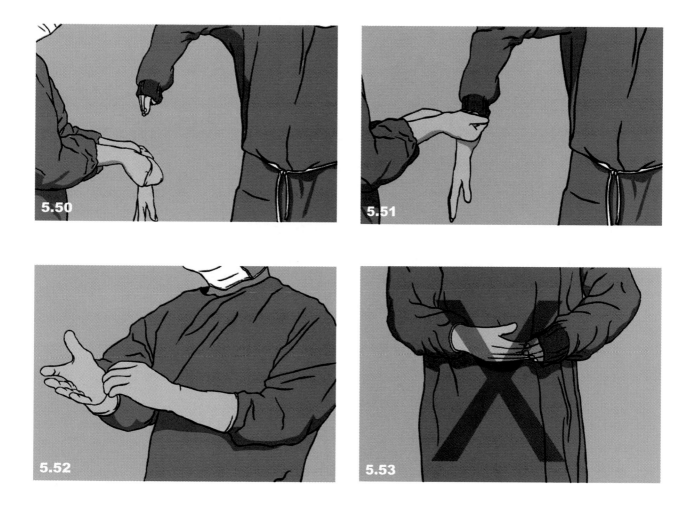

5:1:2:9 Removal of the Contaminated Gown and Glove

If contamination has occurred, the following technique is used to prevent possible spread of contamination.

a) Removal by oneself:

• Open the back of gown
• Slide the gown over shoulders (Figure 5.54).
• To remove the gloves, grasp the wrist section of each glove with the opposite hand and pull simultaneously (Figures 5.55 - 5.58).

b) Removal with the help of the circulating nurse:

• The circulating nurse grasps the gown in front and pulls it toward him/herself (Figure 5.59).
• The gloves can also be removed by the circulating nurse.(Figure 5.60).

notes...

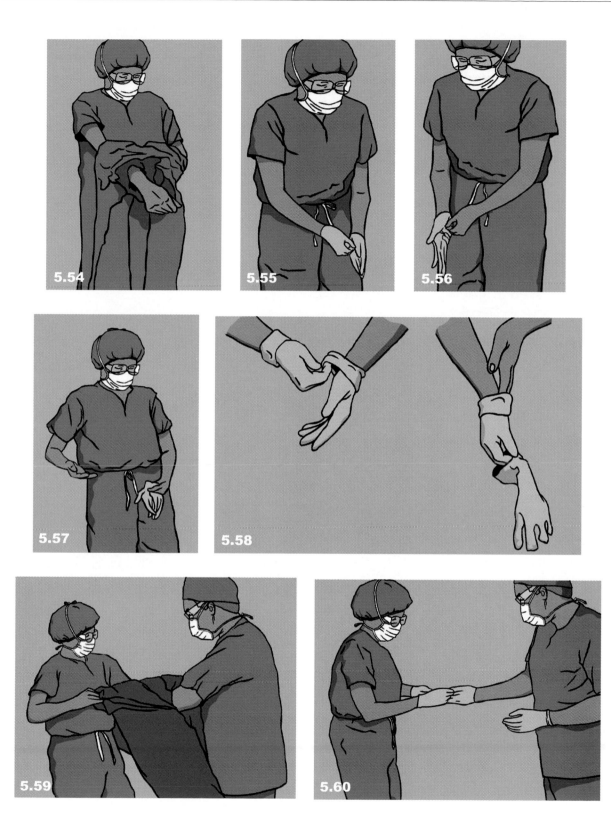

5:1:2:10 Prepping

To prevent the contamination of wounds from microbes that exist in the skin of the patient, the area of the surgical wound is scrubbed with soap and water and then cleaned with antiseptic. This procedure is called prepping. Prepping is performed in an organized fashion drawing a circle or a square around the incision line. The umbilicus may be cleaned of debris by using swabs soaked in anteseptic solution (Figure 5.61). The most important principle for prepping is to start cleaning from the center (line of incision) to the periphery. It is not allowed to bring the gauze from the periphery back to the center even though it is soaked with antiseptic. If there is a need to clean the center again, this is accomplished with the second coating using a new gauze with antiseptic and starting close to the center to the periphery again. The cleaning process can be repeated 2-3 times. Some solutions like proviodine solution must be on the skin for 60 seconds for full effectiveness (Figures 5.62 - 5.66).

NB: Should the prep extend down to the bedline, then one should walk around the OR table, rather than leaning over and contaminating the prepped area.

notes...

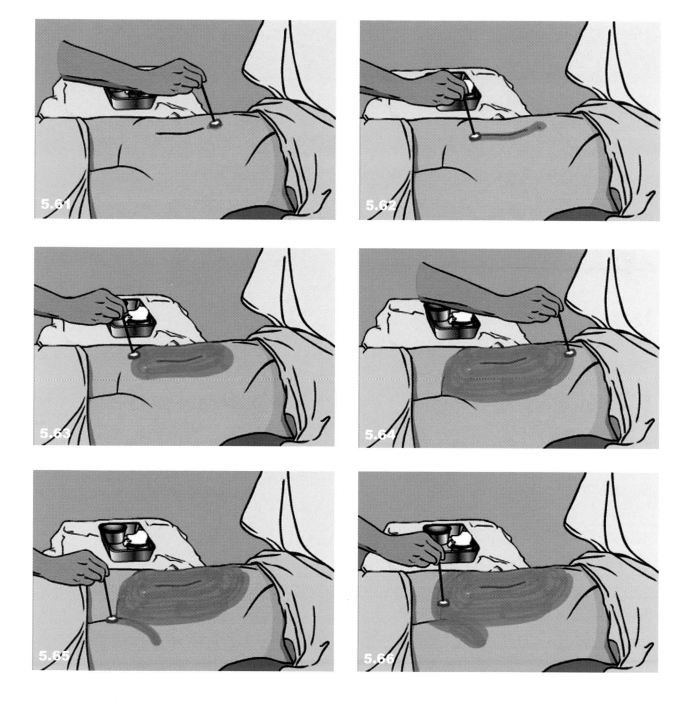

5:1:2:11 Draping

Sterile drapes are used to cover the areas that surround the operation field. Drapes should be placed on the patient without touching the non-sterile areas. The sterile drape should cover the side of the operator first (Figure 5.67) and then the other sides can be covered. In order to avoid touching the non-sterile environment, one can fold the drapes for covering the opposite, up or down sides of the operating field (Figure 5.68). A large drape can be folded from the middle of the operating using the help of a surgical assistant or scrub nurse (Figure 5.69). Care should be taken to protect the gloved hand by making a cuff with the drape around the sterile fingers (Figures 5.70 a & 5.70 b). Once the sterile drape is in place it should not be adjusted. If minor adjustment is required, it should be from the centre toward the periphery, not from the periphery to the centre.

NB: Each hospital may have its own policies and procedures regarding sterile technique. Understanding the basic principles of asepsis will help one to adapt.

notes...

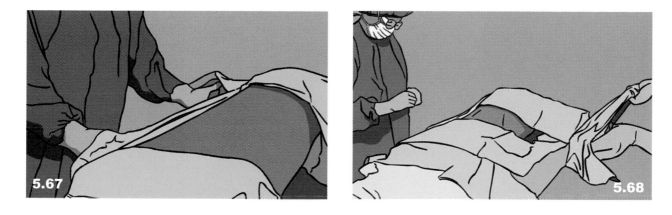

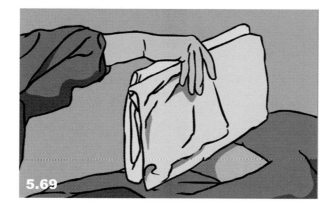

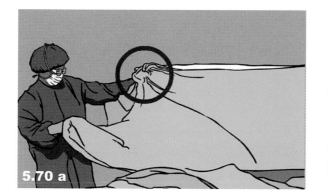

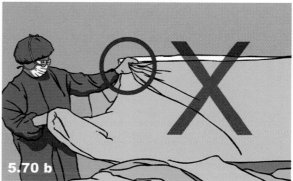

5:1:2:12 Operating room conduct

When in the operating room:

• DO NOT come close to the sterile operating table, scrubbed surgeon, assistant or nurses while observing a procedure.
• DO NOT stand any closer than a foot away from the sterile field.
• DO NOT talk or distract the operating team.
• DO NOT try to be helpful to sterile team. Do not grab or touch things that are unfamiliar unless specifically asked to do so.
• DO NOT assume improper position (Figure 5.71 - 5.73) when scrubbed. Proper position is illustrated in Figure 5.74.
• DO NOT change position face-to-back. Always change position back-to-back (Figure 5.75).

notes...

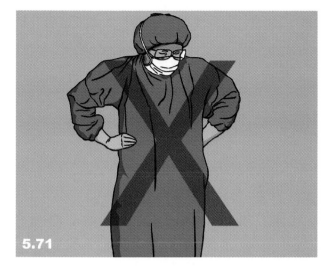

5.71

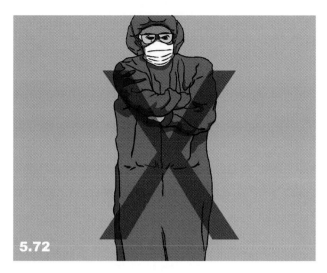

5.72

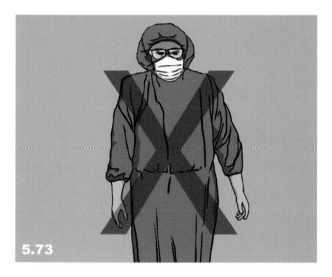

5.73

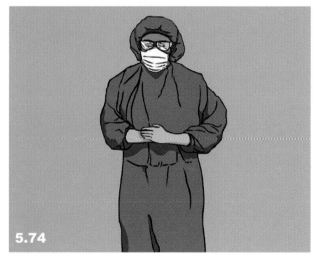

5.74

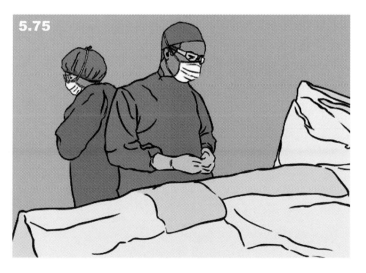

5.75

5:1:3 Prevention of Contamination from Implantation

For prevention of contamination with implantable materials, such as sutures and other bioprosthesis, special sterilizing techniques are used. The sterilization of implantable materials is very important. Due to the structure of materials and the length of time that material is implanted in the body of the patient, it is very complicated to achieve total sterility. Therefore, most of these materials are sterilized and packaged at the production site with specific sterilization techniques such as gamma radiation, gas sterilization, or other specific techniques. Figures 5.76 (sutures), 5.77 (graft conduit) and 5.78 (porcine valve) demonstrate some examples of implantable materials that need extra sterilization caution.

5:2 General Principles

The entire hospital environment must be protected from colonization of virulent strains of bacteria that have a profound effect in the outcome of surgical wounds. Hospital cross-infection is a term used for endemic, in-hospital strains of bacteria that are resistant to many antimicrobial drugs. These organisms include Staphylococcus aureus, Streptococcus, E. coli, Proteus vulgaris and Pseudomonas aeruginosa. Poor hospital management of aseptic precautions lead to higher incidences of wound infections, as well as pneumonitis and septicemia in infants and elderly patients. In order to avoid hospital cross-infection, rules must be strictly enforced in the surgical world of a hospital.

The hospital should have a Surgical Infection Control Program with a Hospital Infection Committee to set up and enforce the following general rules:

a) All significant infections must be reported immediately
b) Infected wounds must be cultured and examined for antibiotic sensitivity
c) Isolation of patients with communicable infections
d) Implementation of aseptic techniques in the operating room
e) Post-operative care of infected open wounds by special dressings, etc.
f) Hand washing before and after contact with patients
g) Personnel with acute, chronic and carrier bacterial status must be detected and excluded from patient contact during treatment, and replaced if it is difficult to fully cure the person
h) Every significant infection should be investigated for the possible detection of source.

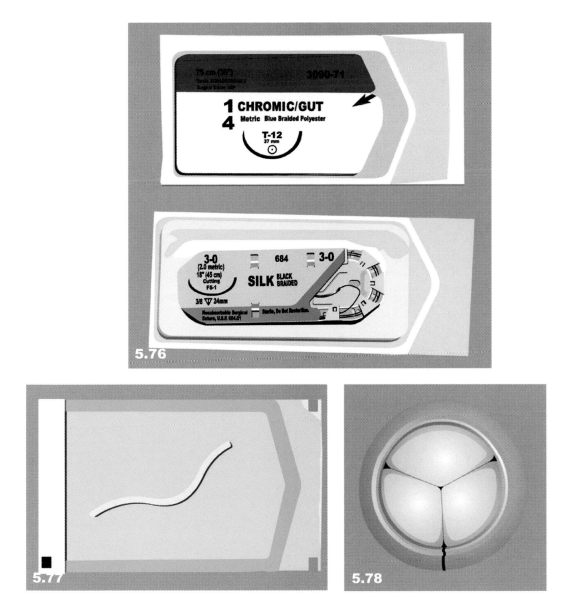

5.76

5.77

5.78

Chapter 6

Basic Surgical Procedures

Chapter 6		Contents	Page

It is difficult to define the basic surgical procedures and to have a general consensus as to which surgical procedures are to be considered basic. This chapter describes procedures that are simple to perform and that may be performed by family physicians or any MD regardless of their specialty. In this chapter, the theoretical basis of the procedures including indications, contraindications and complications are not discussed. This chapter describes the anatomical considerations and the techniques for the performance of the procedures.

It is important to remember that the first, and most important, step in any surgical procedure is preparation. This includes gathering and opening supplies such as instruments, solution for prepping the skin, garbage can, etc. Both the patient and the doctor should be positioned appropriately. Procedures are not always simply done on the first attempt, therefore both the doctor and the patient should be comfortable and prepared for repeated attempts. The last step in any procedure is to clean up, and in particular, to safely dispose of all sharps in a sharps container.

6:1 Venipuncture

The most common site of venipuncture is the antecubital vein. Venipuncture can also be performed in any other superficial vein in the upper or lower extremities.

6:1:1 Technique

a) Apply a tourniquet on the arm proximal to the puncture site, sufficiently tight to interfere with the venous return, but not restricting arterial flow. To aid in filling the veins, the patient can open and close his/her hand. Slapping the arm over the vein is also helpful (Figure 6.1 a and b).

b) Insert the needle bevel up, first through the skin parallel to the vein. Then change the direction so that the needle is pushed against the side of the vein, with the bevel facing away, in order to enter the vein (Figure 6.2 a - 6.2 b).

c) When the needle is inside the vein, blood shows within the syringe. With a further change in direction, advance the needle into the venous cavity (Figure 6.3 a - 6.3 b). If a Teflon catheter is used for the purpose of IV infusion, advance the catheter, take the needle out, and connect the infusion set (Figure 6.4).

d) Fix the needle with adhesive plaster by crossing and wrapping the needle at the hub before the junction with the IV set (Figure 6.5).

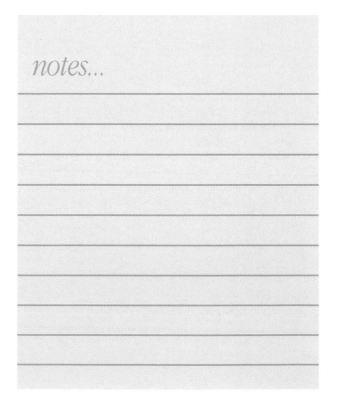

notes...

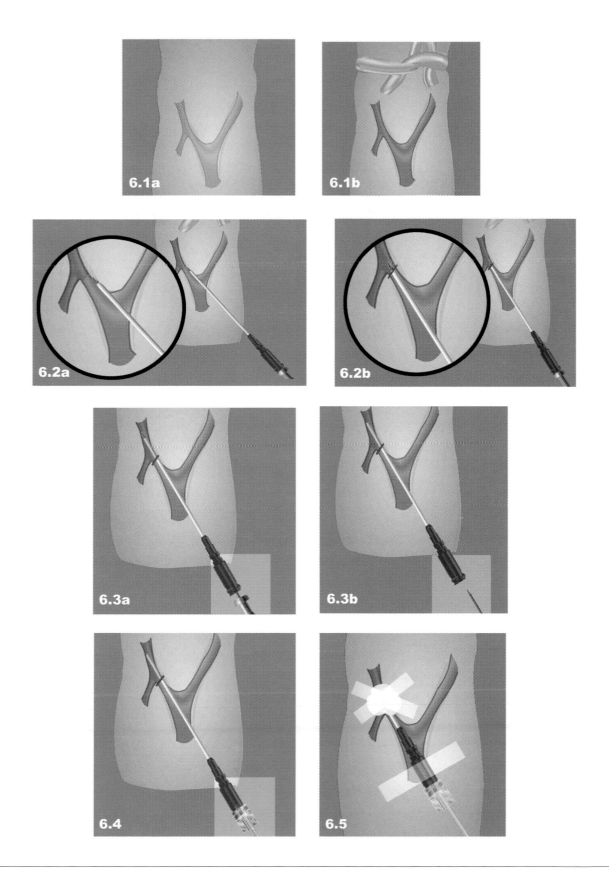

6:2 Arterial Puncture

Arterial puncture is performed for blood gas analysis, arterial blood pressure monitoring or delivery of drugs and contrast materials. Arterial puncture is best performed on femoral or radial arteries.

6:2:1 Technique

a) Provide aseptic conditions.

b) Palpate the pulse on the artery (location of the artery) (Figures 6.6 a - 6.6 b).

c) Insert the needle above the artery through the skin with bevel up, just under the palpated pulse. The femoral vein is located medially and the femoral artery is lateral to the vein in the femoral triangle just beneath the inguinal ligament (Figure 6.7).

d) When blood appears in the needle, withdraw from the artery to the syringe (Figure 6.8). In the case of monitoring, push a Teflon catheter into the artery.

e) Fix the catheter with adhesive plaster or a suture (Figure 6.9).

f) After withdrawal of the needle, press the site of the puncture for at least three minutes (Figure 6.10).

notes...

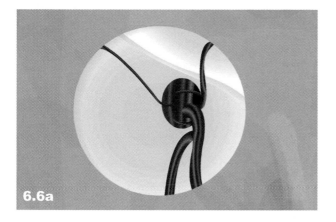

6.6a

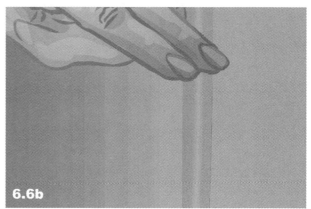

6.6b

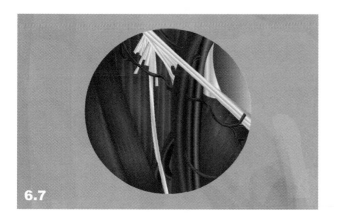

6.7

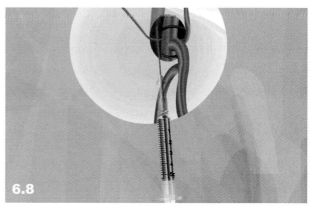

6.8

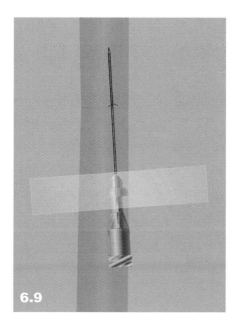

6.9

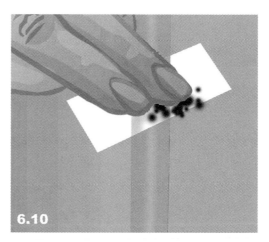

6.10

6:3 Venous Cutdown (cannulation)

Venous cutdown is performed when a suitable vein is not available or percutaneous insertion is impossible. The most commonly used veins for cutdown are the greater saphenous vein, basilic vein, cephalic vein, brachial vein and the external jugular vein.

6:3:1 Topographical Anatomy

a) The Greater Saphenous Vein

The greater saphenous vein is the longest vein in the human body and its pathway is almost subcutaneous. In the region of the popliteal fossa, the saphenous vein runs deep in the fat tissue, it then ascends medially into the thigh and lies more superficially such as in the malleolar and knee-tibial region. The greater saphenous vein can be reached for venous cutdown at the following locations:

i) Medial Malleolus. At this location, the vein lies adjacent to the periosteum and is accompanied by the saphenous nerve, which if transected, causes sensory loss in a small area along the medial aspect of the foot. At this location, the vein can be exposed with minimal blunt dissection. This superficial, isolated, and predictable location has made this site a classical cutdown site for the "great" (long) saphenous vein

(Figure 6.11 a).

ii) Medial Aspect of the Knee. At this location, the saphenous vein lies superficially. A cutdown performed 1 to 4 cm below the knee and immediately posterior to the tibia is described in older pediatric literature. However, this site of cutdown is now seldomly used. Disadvantages of this technique include kinking of the line as the knee is flexed and risk of injury to associated structures. Improper incision may cause injury of the following structures: the saphenous vein and the saphenous branch of the genicular artery (Figure 6.11 b).

iii) Fossa Ovalis. In the thigh, the saphenous vein ascends from the medial aspects of the knee (above popliteal fossa) toward the femoral triangle. Proximally, it enters the fossa ovalis and joins the femoral vein. The outside diameter of the great saphenous vein in this region is 4-5 mm. Lateral to the great saphenous vein lies the lateral femoral cutaneous vein, which has a smaller diameter (2-3 mm) and is therefore easily distinguishable from the great saphenous vein through the cutdown operation (Figures 6.11 c and 6.6 a).

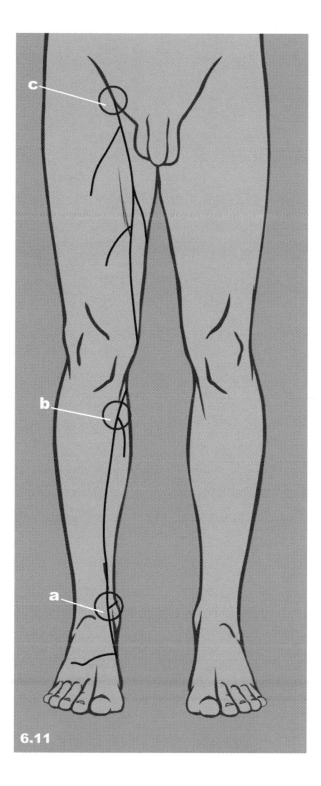

6.11

b) The Basilic Vein

The basilic vein is a preferred site for a venous cutdown in the upper extremity.

At the mid-forearm level, the basilic vein crosses anterolaterally and is consistently found 1-2 cm lateral to the medical epicondyle on the anterior surface of the upper arm. The basilic vein continues proximally, occupying a superficial position between the biceps and pronator teres muscles. The basilic vein is generally cannulated at the antecubital fossa 2 cm above and 2-3 cm lateral to the medial epicondyle (Figure 6.12a).

c) The Cephalic Vein

The cephalic vein is also an appropriate site for a venisection in the upper extremity because of its large diameter and superficial location.

In the antecubital fossa, it lies subcutaneously, just lateral to the midline, and then ascends in the upper arm, overlying the lateral aspect of the biceps muscle. At the shoulder, the cephalic vein lies in the deltopectoral groove. Just below the clavicle, it passes deep to end in the axillary vein (Figure 6.12 b).

d) The Brachial Veins

The brachial veins are small, paired vessels lying on either side of the brachial artery (Figure 6.13). These vessels are not superficial and will not accommodate a large cannulae. Their most superficial location is 1-2 cm above the antecubital fossa just medial to the biceps muscle. Palpation of the brachial pulse serves as a useful landmark but the artery may be inadvertently cannulated in patients with low blood pressure. Additionally, there is the risk of injury to the closely associated median nerve. This site may be acceptable when access time and vessel size are not critical factors. In addition, the metacarpal veins (Figure 6.14) are also used frequently for venous access.

e) The External Jugular Vein

The external jugular vein begins below the angle of the mandible formed by confluence of the posterior auricular and retromandibular veins. It descends posterolaterally across the surface of the sternocleidomastoid muscle and then pierces the fascia to join the subclavian vein deep to the clavicular head of this muscle. The greater auricular nerve, which supplies sensation to the external ear, travels parallel to the external jugular vein (Figure 6.15-6.16).

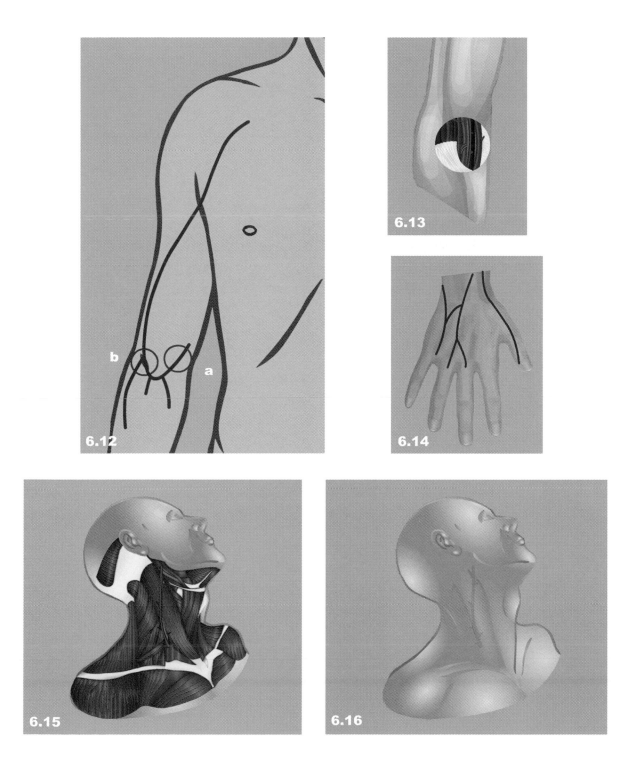

6.12

6.13

6.14

6.15

6.16

6:3:2 Technique

a) Clean the area with antiseptics.

b) Infiltrate anesthesia around the vein.

c) Make a transverse incision perpendicular to the target vein (Figure 6.17).

d) Anteroposterior projection

   - Skin

   - Subcutaneous tissue

e) Dissect the vein from surrounding tissue (Figure 6.18 - 6.21).

f) Pass two ties around the area of the vein designated for cutdown, one proximally, one distally (Figures 6.22 - 6.23).

g) Ligate the distal tie (Figure 6.24).

NB: Remember that the superficial veins are located at the subcutaneous layer. The search for the vein should be performed in the subcutaneous fat. If muscle or other deep structures are exposed, the dissection is too deep.

notes...

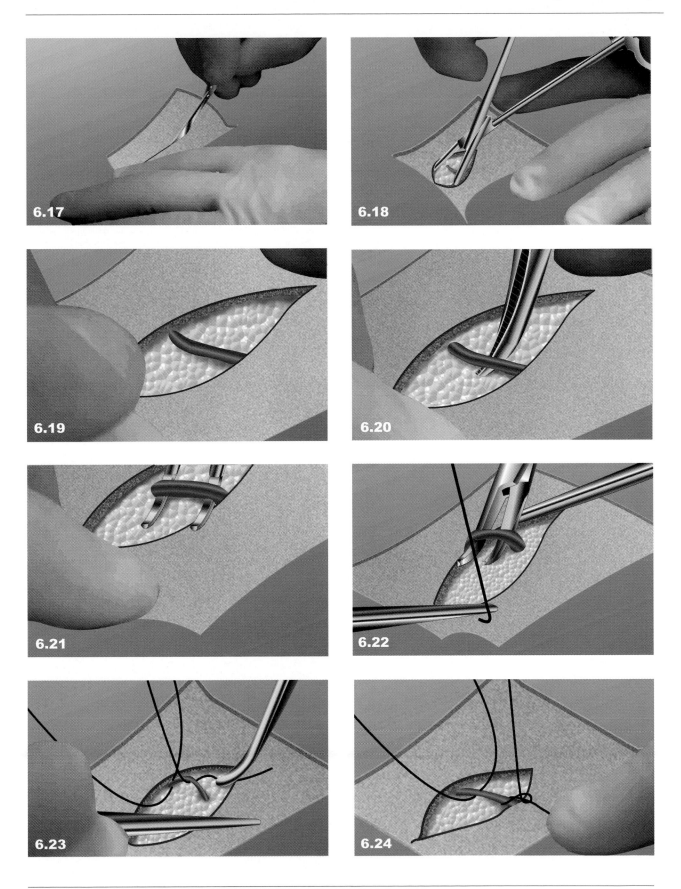

h) Make a "V" shaped incision in the vein or insert a Teflon cannula directly (Figure 6.25).

i) Insert the cannula proximally. Insertion of the cannula can be performed from inside the wound (Figure 6.26) or from outside the wound (Figure 6.27).

j) Ligate the proximal tie over the cannula (Figure 6.28).

k) Remove the needle (Figure 6.29).

l) Connect the cannula and needle to the system (Figure 6.30).

m) Test the cannula by running the fluid.

n) Close the wound with interrupted sutures (Figure 6.31).

o) Secure the cannula with an air knot (Figure 6.32).

p) Apply sterile dressings.

NB: Cannulation of the vein from outside the wound is preferred. In this case the long-term presence of the needle will not interfere with the wound healing. It is important to secure the needle with the air knot as it will prevent the needle from coming out.

notes...

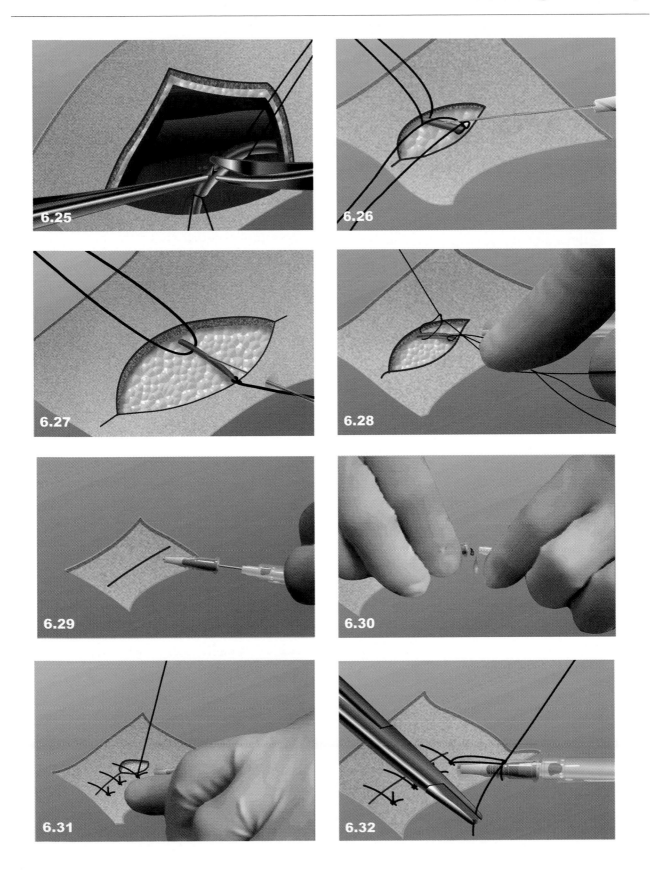

6:4 Subclavian Catheterization

The subclavian vein is used for central venous catheterization. The popularity of central venous catheterization has grown rapidly in recent years. The development of sophisticated monitoring techniques, transvenous pacemaker devices, total parenteral nutrition, and emergency resuscitation protocols have created a need for rapid and reliable methods of central venous access. Peripheral venous sites can be used but the veins may be collapsed, thrombosed, buried in subcutaneous fat or difficult to locate. The subclavian vein has a predictable relationship to easily identifiable landmarks and can be cannulated within minutes.

Due to potential complications such as infection, sepsis, pneumothorax and others, subclavian catheterization is considered to be a surgical procedure. This should be indicated to the patient and a strict aseptic approach is recommended.

6:4:1 Topographical Anatomy

The subclavian vein begins as a continuation of the axillary vein at the outer edge of the first rib. It joins the internal jugular vein to become the innominate vein 3-4 cm proximally. It has a diameter of 10-20 mm and is valveless. After crossing the first rib, the vein lies posteriorly to the medial third of the clavicle. It is only in this area that there is an intimate association between the clavicle and the subclavian vein. The costoclavicular ligament lies anterior and inferior to the subclavian vein and the fascia that is contiguous to this ligament invests the vessel. Posterior to the vein, separating it from the subclavian artery, lies the anterior scalene muscle, which has the thickness of 10-15 mm. The phrenic nerve passes over the anterior surface of the scalene muscle and runs immediately behind the junction of the subclavian and internal jugular veins. The thoracic duct (on the left) and the lymphatic duct (on the right) pass over the anterior scalene muscle and enter the subclavian vein near its junction with the internal jugular vein. Superior and posterior to the subclavian artery lies the brachial plexus. The dome of the left lung may extend above the first rib, however the right lung does not extend this high (Figures 6.33 - 6.38).

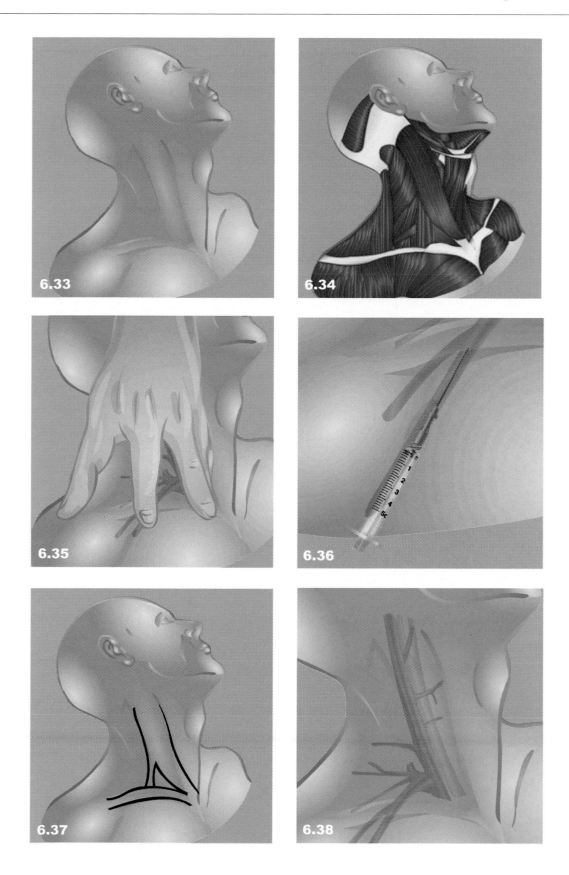

6.33

6.34

6.35

6.36

6.37

6.38

6:4:2 Technique

a) Place the patient in the Trendelenburg position with a rolled towel between the shoulder blades.

b) Prep and drape the area.

c) Landmarks:
- lateral - the lateral aspect of the clavicle
- medial - the sternal notch.

d) Place the thumb on the lateral landmark and the middle finger on the medial landmark, the index finger will fall at the subclavian vein where the needle should be inserted (Figure 6.39).

e) Anterior -Posterior projection
- Skin
- Subcutaneous tissue, clavipectoral fascia
- Pectoral major muscle (clavicular part)
- Subclavian vein

f) Anesthetize the skin and insert the needle (16 gauge) beneath the clavicle with the bevel down. Advance the needle parallel to the bed with the tip directed toward the suprasternal notch. Maintain constant suction on the syringe while moving it forward (Figure 6.40 - 6.41).

g) When blood appears in the syringe, disconnect the syringe, withdraw the needle and insert a J wire through the Teflon catheter left in place, to the superior vena cava (Figure 6.42).

h) Withdraw the catheter and insert an introducer with a catheter into the vein through a 1-2 cm skin incision adjacent to the J-wire (Figure 6.43).

i) Connect an IV set to the catheter, or use the port for other intravenous procedures.

j) Fix the catheter with a suture to the skin and apply an aseptic dressing (Figure 6.44).

notes...

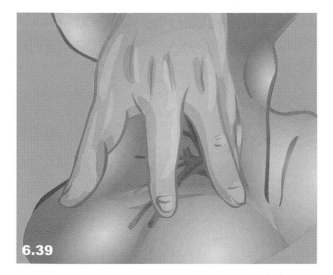

6.39

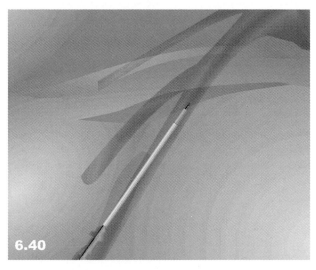

6.40

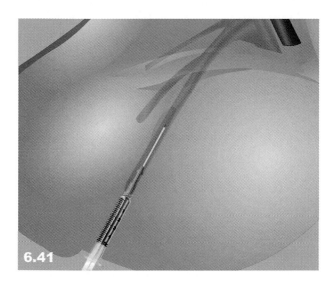

6.41

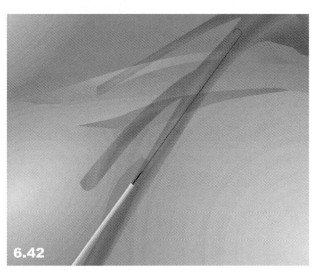

6.42

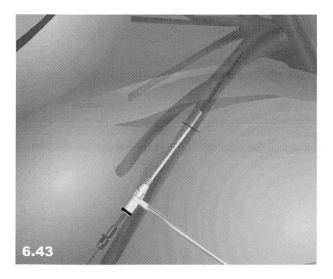

6.43

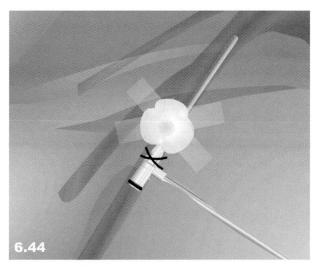

6.44

6:5 Internal Jugular Vein (IJV)

6:5:1 Topographical Anatomy

The landmark for the identification of the internal jugular vein (IJV) is the sternocleidomastoid (SCM) triangle (Figure 6.45-6.46). The lateral wall of this triangle is the clavicular head of the SCM muscle, the medial wall is presented by the sternal head of the SCM muscle and the base of the triangle is formed with the clavicle. The IJV is located under the medial border of the clavicular head (lateral border) of the SCM muscle. The carotid artery is located deeper and at the medial border, i.e. sternal head of the SCM muscle. In order to identify the triangle, the patient must be awake. The right IJV is preferred as it leads directly into the superior vena cava.

The patient should be in a 15° Trendelenberg's position, with the neck extended and turned sharply to the left. When the patient lifts his/her head thereby tensing the muscle, the triangle borders are identified (Figure 6.46). The point of venous puncture is the apex of the SCM triangle which is identified as the junction of the clavicular head and the sternal head of the muscle approximately 1.5-2 inches above the clavicle and lateral to the carotid pulse.

6:5:2 Technique

a) Position the patient as above. Prepare and drape the neck in sterile fashion.

b) Raise a skin wheal with local anesthetic at the apex of the SCM triangle.

c) Locate the vein with a 14 gauge needle on a 5 ml syringe. Advance the needle in the caudal direction at a 30° angle to the skin under the lateral head of the muscle while aspirating on the syringe (Figure 6.47).

d) Remove the syringe and the needle, and introduce a J-wire into the IJV via a Teflon catheter left in the vein (Figure 6.48).

e) After the J-wire is well advanced into the IJV, remove the catheter.

f) A 1-2 mm cut is made in the skin adjacent to the guidewire with the tip of a #11 scalpel blade.

• Pass a dilator over the guidewire to dilate a tract for insertion of the catheter (Figure 6.49).

g) Remove the dilator and pass the catheter, with introducer, over the guidewire. Remove the guidewire.

h) Remove the introducer and connect the catheter to the intravenous tubing or flush with heparinized saline (Figure 6.50).

i) Suture the catheter in place and apply a sterile dressing.

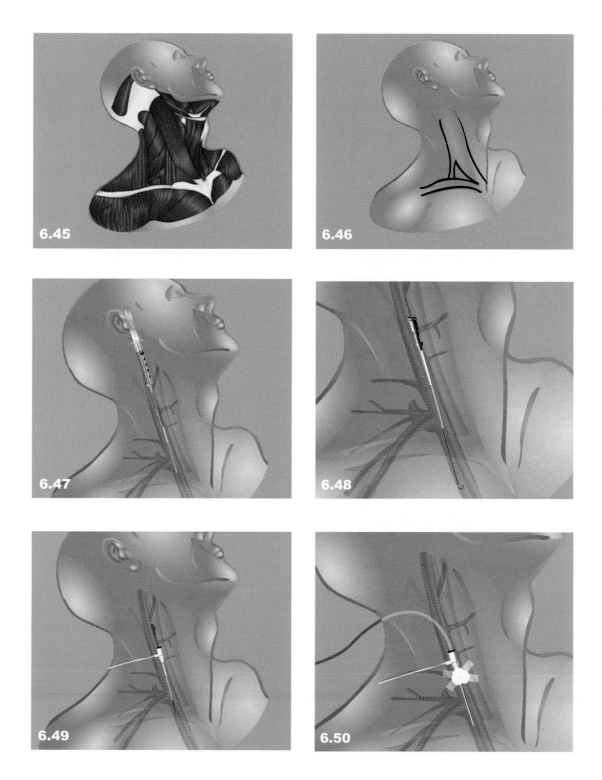

6.45

6.46

6.47

6.48

6.49

6.50

6:6 External Jugular Vein (EJV)

6:6:1 Topographical Anatomy

The external jugular vein (EJV) is rarely used as an alternative to the IJV when it is difficult to access the IJV. The landmark for the EJV is the body of the SCM muscle. The EJV descends posterolaterally across the surface of the SCM muscle. The vein may be easily reached at the middle part of the posterior border of the SCM muscle (Figure 6.51-6.52).

Place the patient in a 15° Trendelenberg's position with the neck extended and turned sharply to the left. The vein is usually visible on the surface of the SCM muscle. It is extremely difficult to have central access via the EJV, therefore a J-wire catheterization technique should be used.

N.B.: Some practitioners do not find the EJV to be a good route for insertion of the Swan-Ganz catheter.

6:6:2 Technique

a) Position the patient as above. Prepare and drape the neck in sterile fashion.

b) Raise a skin wheal with local anesthetic at the surface of the SCM muscle above the apex of the SCM triangle.

c) Enter the EJV with a 5 ml syringe using a 14 gauge needle with over the needle Teflon catheter. Advance the needle while aspirating.

d) Introduce a J-wire through the Teflon catheter after the needle is removed. Rotate the J-wire past venous valvular obstructions into the central circulation (Figure 6.53).

e) Make a 1-2 mm cut in the skin adjacent to the guidewire with the tip of a #11 scalpel blade.

f) Pass a dilator over the guidewire to dilate a tract for insertion of the catheter.

g) Remove the dilator and pass the catheter, with introducer, over the guidewire (Figures 6.54 - 6.55).

h) Remove the introducer and connect the catheter to the intravenous tubing or flush with heparinized saline (Figure 6.56).

i) Suture the catheter in place and apply a sterile dressing.

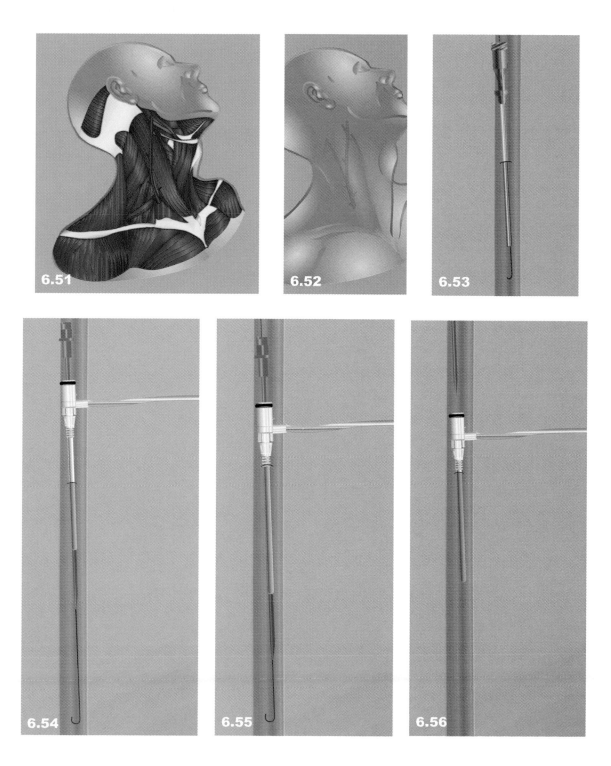

6.51

6.52

6.53

6.54

6.55

6.56

6:7 Swan-Ganz Catheter

The Swan-Ganz catheter is considered to be one of the major advances in hemodynamic monitoring. For adults, Swan-Ganz catheters are available in 5-Fr. and 7-Fr. sizes. The catheter has two pressure lumens with one located at the tip and the second about 30 cm back from the tip. It also has an inflatable balloon and a thermistor located behind the balloon. The lumen at the tip measures systolic, diastolic and mean pulmonary artery pressure (PAP). The second lumen, 30 cm back from the tip, measures the central venous pressure (CVP). When the balloon is inflated inside the pulmonary artery, it occludes the blood flow and thus the catheter is capable of measuring the pulmonary capillary wedge pressure (PCWP). The PCWP can be used as an indirect measurement of the left atrial pressure (LAP) due to its good correlation with the LAP. Thus PCWP can be used as a measure of left ventricular filling pressure.

6:7:1 Technique

The Swan-Ganz catheter can be introduced by a variety of techniques:

a) Open technique (venous cutdown)

• Cleanse the area with antiseptic solution
• Infiltrate the skin over the vein with 0.5% lidocaine.
• Make a transverse incision perpendicular to the site of the venous cutdown (Figure 6.57). The antecubital fossae was the original site for Swan-Ganz catheters but is rarely used at the present time.
• Isolate the vein by blunt dissection from the surrounding tissue (Figure 6.58 - 6.59).
• Pass two ties around the area designated for cutdown, one proximally and one distally, and ligate the distal tie (Figure 6.60).
• Make a "V" shaped incision in the vein (Figure 6.61).
• Advance the Swan-Ganz catheter through the cutdown into the right atrium (Figure 6.62).

notes...

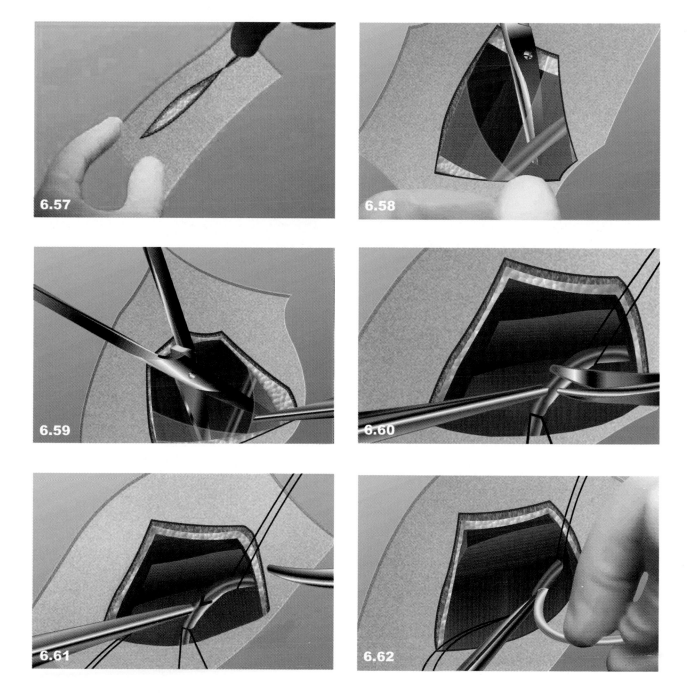

b) Percutaneous technique through a central vein access such as IJV access (Figure 6.63) (see IJV for detailed description).

In both techniques, the Swan-Ganz catheter is passed to the right atrium and the location of the catheter is judged via a high-frequency pressure transducer connected to a monitor. In general, the catheter is advanced with the balloon inflated ("floated" in), and withdrawn with the balloon deflated, to avoid damage to the cardiac valves (Figure 6.64).

Steps:

• Fill the Swan-Ganz catheter with fluid, examine the balloon with air and attach to the transducer (Figure 6.65 - 6.66).
• Pass the catheter through the sheath or venous cutdown into the superior vena cava and advance about 20 cm into the superior vena cava. At this time the monitor should show atrial tracing with pressure of about 6/0 mmHg. This indicates that the catheter is in the right atrium (Figure 6.67).
• Put 1 cc of air into the balloon to allow it to float into the right ventricle. The indication for the location of the catheter is change in the character of the pressure tracing, as well as the values (30/5 mmHg, Figure 6.68).
• In the right ventricle, put 1.5 cc of air into the balloon to completely cover the tip of the catheter in an effort to reduce complications such as ventricular arrhythmias. (Figure 6.68).
• Advance the catheter further into the pulmonary artery. The inflated balloon will be carried with the flow to the pulmonary artery. In the pulmonary artery the character of the pressure waves is changed again, with values of about 25/10 mmHg (Figure 6.69).
• When the pulmonary artery tracing is absorbed, advance the catheter further up until the PCWP is observed (Figure 6.70). The monitor at this time shows a straight line with values of about 12/1 mmHg.
• Deflate the balloon to observe the pulmonary artery tracing again. Values should return to about 25/10 mmHg (Figure 6.71).
• Determine cardiac output by thermal dilution technique. This can also be obtained with a Swan Ganz catheter.
• Inject a 2 ml aliquot of cold (0°-2°C) 5% dextrose in water to the proximal lumen of the catheter. The cardiac output computer can calculate the cardiac output via the thermal dilution method.

NB: The most common site of long term and efficient venous access is the internal jugular vein.

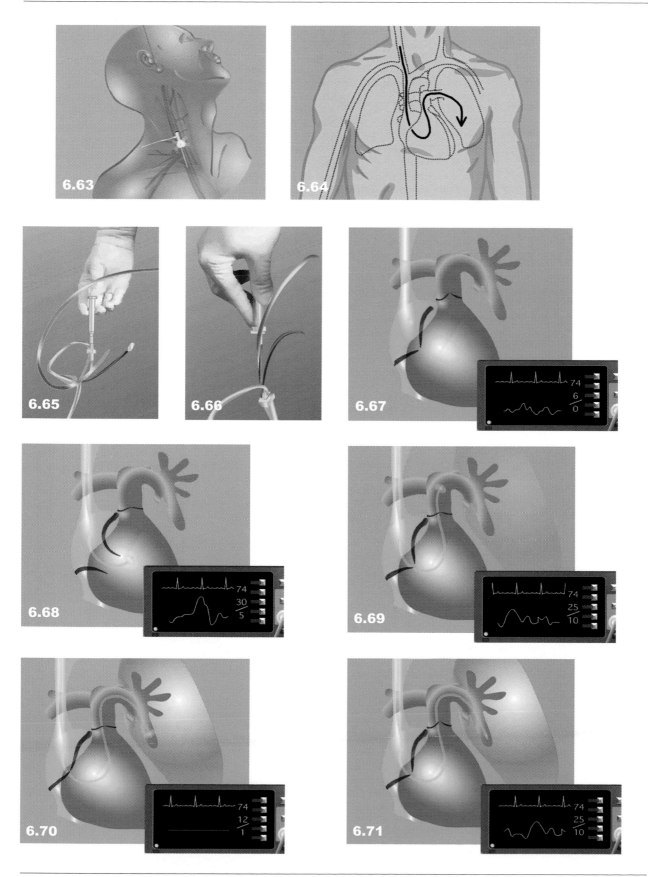

6.63

6.64

6.65

6.66

6.67

6.68

6.69

6.70

6.71

6:8 Arterial Cannulation

Arterial cannulation is mainly used for direct monitoring of blood pressure, cardiac and coronary artery catheterization, multiple arterial blood gas measurement, selected anesthetic procedures and others.

The preferred sites for arterial cannulation are:

• Radial artery
• Ulnar artery
• Brachial or axillary arteries
• Femoral artery (Figure 6.72-6.73)
• Dorsalis pedis artery

a) Percutanous Cannulation Technique

• Lay the patient in the supine position.
• Raise a skin wheal over the artery with local anesthesia.
• Prepare the site of cannulation with antiseptic solution.
• Identify the pulse (Figure 6.74).
• Insert a 14-16 gauge needle with a Teflon catheter into the artery (Figure 6.75). Once the needle is in the artery, advance the catheter and remove the needle. Connect the catheter with the arterial line to the pressure transducer and monitoring system.

When Atrial Catheterization is Required:

• Introduce a J-wire through the Teflon catheter into the artery and remove the Teflon sheet (Figure 6.76).
• Make a 1-2 mm cut in the skin adjacent to the guidewire with the tip of an #11 scalpel blade.
• Pass a dilator over the guidewire to dilate a tract for insertion of the catheter.
• Remove the dilator and pass the catheter, with introducer inserted through it, over the guidewire as described in venous catheterization (Figure 6.77).
• The port is fixed and is ready to be used for the introduction of the long special catheter.

NB: The most common site of arterial puncture is the radial and femoral arteries.

notes...

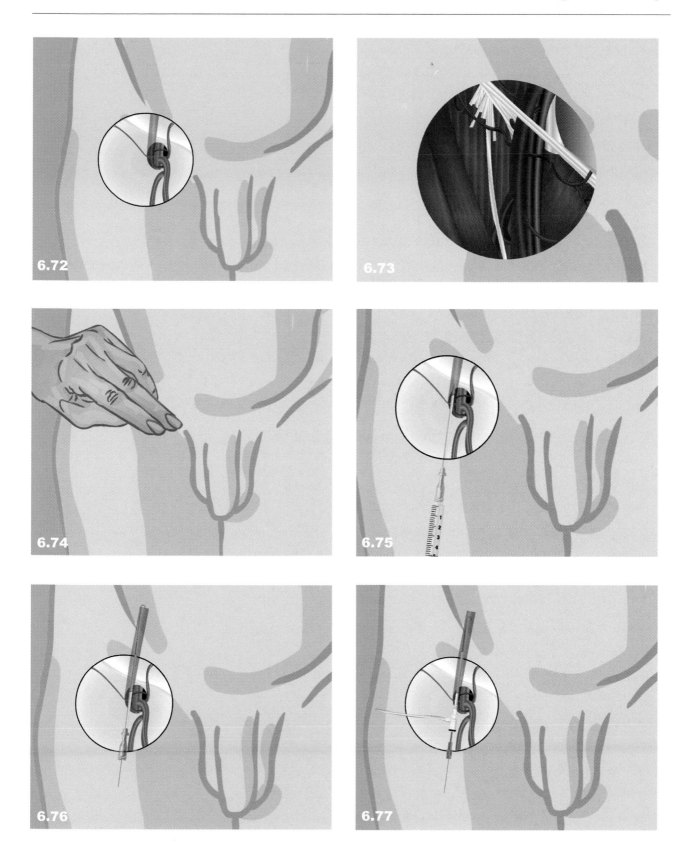

6.72

6.73

6.74

6.75

6.76

6.77

b) Direct Cannulation Technique

The direct technique is usually used in experimental conditions or for intra-operative procedures.

• For the direct technique, dissect the artery and pass two ties or umbilical tapes proximally and distally to the area designated for catheterization (Figure 6.78-6.79).
• Pass the ties or umbilical tapes through a rubber tube (Figure 6.80-6.81).
• Pull the distal snare down and secure with the help of a mosquito clamp in order to close the artery and interrupt the flow distally (Figure 6.82).
• Introduce a 14-16 gauge needle with a Teflon sheet into the artery proximally (Figure 6.83).
• Pull the second snare on the top of the catheter to interrupt the leakage around the catheter.
• Connect the catheter to the pressure line (Figure 6.84).
• Tie and secure the line and the catheter with a silk tie to the distal rubber tube (Figure 6.85).

NB: Direct technique for arterial cannulation is used very rarely. It is mostly an experimental procedure.

notes...

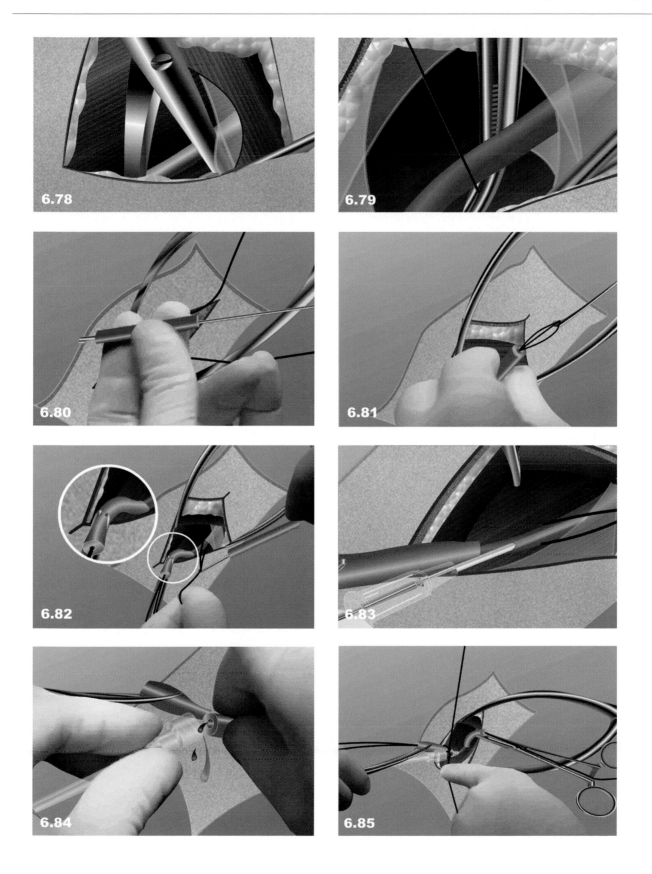

6:9 Techniques For Airway Access

The correct terminology for airway access is tracheostomy. This terminology is derived from "trachea arteria", a Greek word for "rough artery", and "tome" meaning cut; hence the terminology "tracheotomy". The word "tracheostomy" is derived from the Greek word "stoma" meaning mouth. This terminology should not be used unless a tube is planned as a permanent opening. In some older lectures, the words "upper" and "lower" tracheotomy are used. At the present time, tracheotomy is used only for "lower tracheotomy." The new nomenclature for an upper tracheotomy is cricothyroidotomy.

6:9:1 Topographical Anatomy

The sternocleidomastoid or sternomastoid muscle divides the neck into an anterior triangle and posterior triangle. Tracheotomy is performed in the lower part of the anterior triangle (Figure 6.86).

6:9:2 Cricothyroidotomy

This procedure is performed only in emergency cases for rapid airway access; it should be converted to a tracheotomy as soon as possible.

- Place patient in supine position with neck extended. Prepare and drape anterior part of the neck (Figure 6.86).
- Infiltrate locally with xylocaine 1:100,000 epinephrine or general anesthesia (Figure 6.87).
- Stabilize the thyroid cartilage with left hand (thumb and index finger); make a horizontal skin incision over the lower half of the cricothyroid membrane (Figure 6.88).
- Carefully incise the cricothyroid membrane and, with the help of a blunt instrument such as arterial clamp or handle of the scalpel, open the airway (Figure 6.89).
- Insert an endotracheal tube of appropriate size through the incision and direct into the trachea (Figure 6.90).
- Inflate the cuff and connect the tube to the respirator; close the wound around the tube with interrupted sutures and fix tube with air knots (Figure 6.91).

NB: In an emergency, sterility is a secondary consideration. One can use any tubular object, such as a pen, to open the airway to outside air.

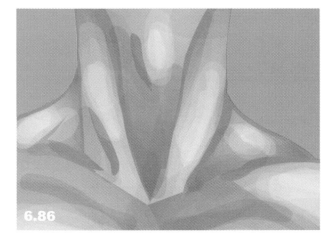

6.86

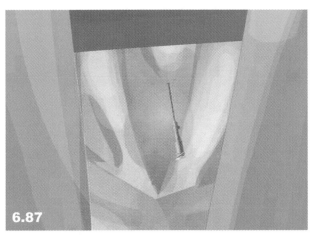

6.87

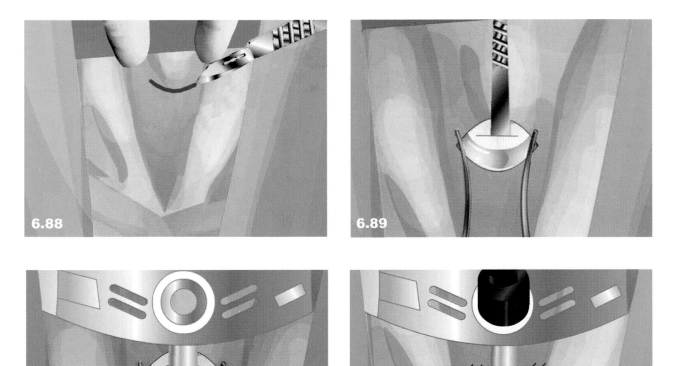

6.88

6.89

6.90

6.91

6:9:3 Tracheotomy (Tracheostomy) Technique

• Place patient in supine position with neck extended. Prepare and drape anterior part of the neck.

• Infiltrate locally with xylocaine 1:100,000 epinephrine or general anesthesia (Figure 6.92).

• Anteroposterior projection

- skin
- superficial fascia and subcutaneous connective tissue
- superficial layer of the deep cervical fascia
- pre-tracheal fascia
- infrahyoid (strap or ribbon) muscles
- pre-tracheal space
- trachea

• Make a horizontal incision in a skin crease about 2.5 cm beneath the cricoid cartilage. A vertical incision is used for urgent cases (Figure 6.93).

• Reach strap muscles and retract laterally from the midline. Continue blunt dissection until the thyroid isthmus is exposed and reflected superiorly (do not cut the isthmus unless the thyroid is large and unavoidable) (Figure 6.94 - 6.95).

• Place two-stay sutures of 2.0 silk in the cartilage on either side of the 3rd tracheal ring (Figure 6.96 - 6.97).

notes...

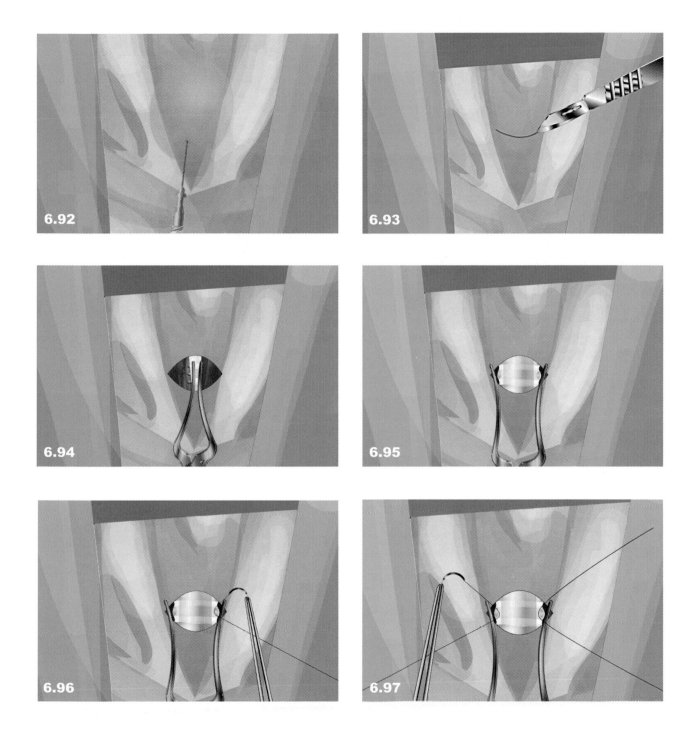

6.92

6.93

6.94

6.95

6.96

6.97

• Make a horizontal incision in the 2nd or 3rd intercartilaginous space (Figure 6.98). Pull tracheal traction sutures at either side of opening in the trachea. Deflate the endotracheal tube and pull up if one is in place, but do not take it out (Figures 6.99 a - 6.99 b).

• Elevate the lower cartilaginous ring with a hook and insert an appropriately sized tracheostomy tube; inflate the cuff and connect to the respirator (Figure 6.100).

• Do not take out the stay sutures. They should be folded inside the wound (Figure 6.101). In case of the accidental removal of the endotrachial tube, they can be used to re-insert the tube.

• Use simple interrupted sutures to close the wound (Figure 6.102-6.103).

NB: Trachiotomy is an urgent or a routine procedure. Therefore strict aseptic laws should be applied. Most patients are intubated- care should be taken when the endotrachial tube is removed and the tracheotomy tube is inserted.

notes...

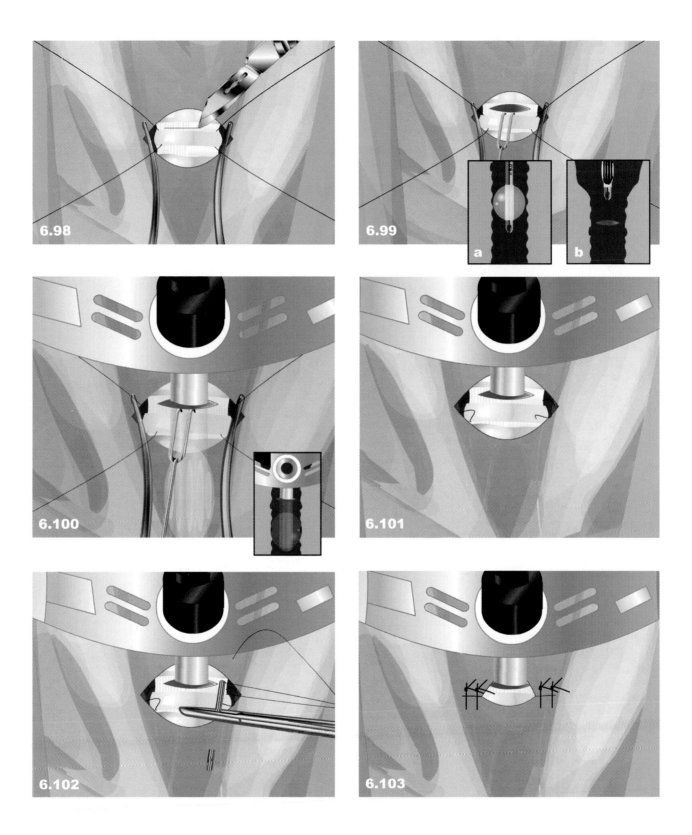

6:10 Thoracocentesis

Thoracocentesis is a surgical procedure performed for the removal of fluid such as exudate, blood or air from the pleural cavity.

6:10:1 Topographical Anatomy

In the intercostal space (between 2nd and 3rd rib) the needle insertion or incision should be made at the upper margin of the rib in order to avoid damage to the neurovascular intercostal bundle (vein, artery, nerve) located in subcostal groove.

• Anteroposterior projection
- 2nd intercostal space anteriorly at the midclavicular line to remove air (Figure 6.104 - 6.105).
- skin
- subcutaneous tissue and fascia (in females, it also includes mammary glands)
- superficial pectoral fascia
- external intercostal fascia
- external intercostal muscle
- internal intercostal muscle
- innermost intercostal muscle
- parietal (costal) pleura
- pleural cavity

• For the removal of fluid, the location is posterior or mid-axillary line on 5th or 6th intercostal space (Figure 6.106).

- skin
- subcutaneous tissue
- latissimus dorsi (for posterior axillary line) and serratus anterior (for mid-axillary line)
- external intercostal fascia
- external intercostal muscle
- internal intercostal muscle
- innermost intercostal muscle
- parietal pleura
- pleural cavity

6:10:2 Needle Aspiration Techniques

a) The patient must be in a comfortable sitting position with hands comfortably lying on a table in front of them.

b) Posterioanterior and lateral x-rays as well as careful percussion are needed to localize the level of fluid or air.

c) Prep and drape using aseptic techniques.

d) Infiltrate with xylocaine (1:10,000 epinephrine).

e) Insert the needle (Figure 6.107-6.108).

f) Attach a three-way stopcock to the needle and connect it to the collecting reservoir. (Figure 1.109). Withdraw with the fluid in the syringe and empty it to the reservoir.

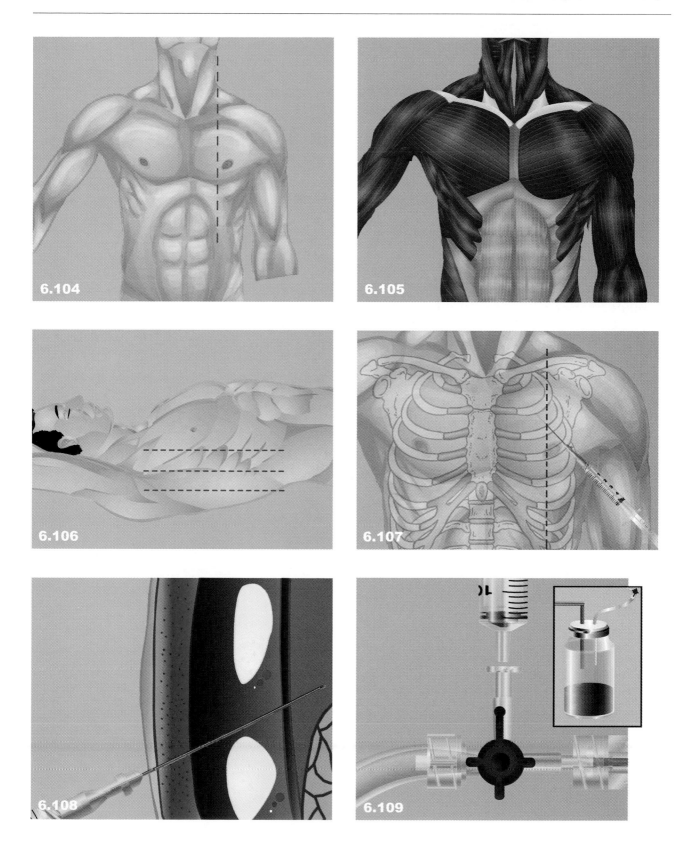

6.104

6.105

6.106

6.107

6.108

6.109

6:10:3 Chest Tube Technique

a) Prepare the area with antiseptic solutions and cover with sterile drapes (Figure 6.110).

b) Infiltrate with local anesthesia, lidocaine 0.5% (1:10,000 epinephrine) (Figure 6.111).

c) Make a small (2-3 cm) incision of the skin and pectoral fascia parallel to the upper section of the ribs with a bayonet-tip scalpel blade at the anatomical landmarks (Figure 6.112 - 6.114).

d) When the ribs are visible or palpable, divide the intercostal muscle with blunt dissection using a heavy and dull instrument such as a Kelly forceps (Figure 6.115). Place the Kelly behind the index finger and above the rib. Open the intercostal muscles separately.

e) Use the index finger to feel the depth of the dissected wound. When the finger touches the parietal pleura, the instrument should be taken away. With the help of the index finger, rupture the pleura and penetrate the chest cavity (Figure 6.116).

f) Move the index finger inside the chest around the wound in order to check for adhesions or other structural barriers (Figure 6.117).

notes...

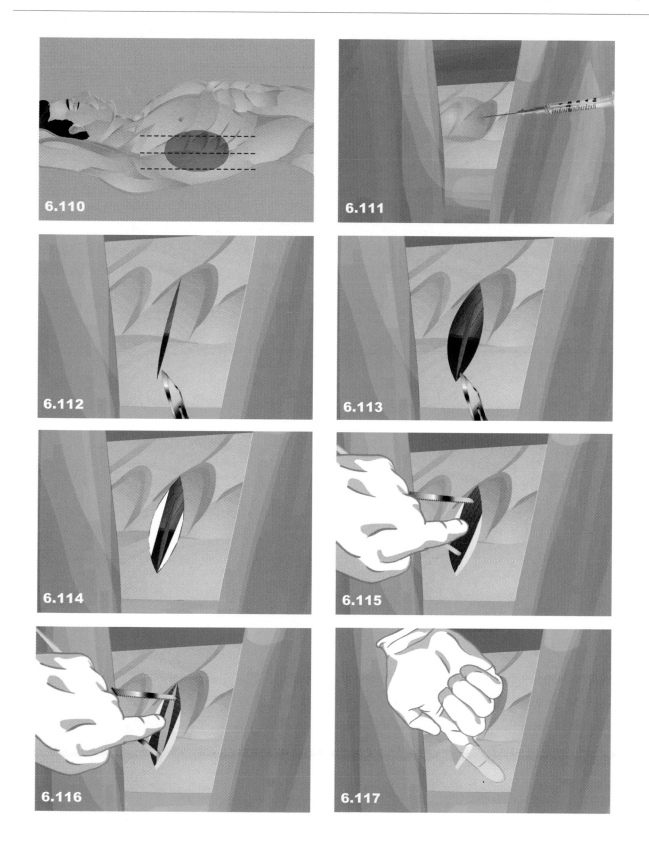

6.110

6.111

6.112

6.113

6.114

6.115

6.116

6.117

g) Insert the chest tube into the chest cavity with the help of hemostats (Figure 6.118 - 6.119). The curve of the hemostst should be parallel to the tube. Once the tube is inside the chest cavity, push the tube posteriorly and medially.

h) Place two vertical mattress sutures on either side of the tube. An untied horizontal mattress suture around the tube is also desirable (Figure 6.120). The latter suture is used to close the wound when the tube is removed.

i) Anchor the tube with the skin suture to prevent the tube from pulling out (Figure 6.120).

j) Connect the chest tube into a double-bottle water-sealed system. The tube in the second bottle should be 1 cm under the water. When the pressure rises more then 1 cm water in the chest, the air or the fluid could bubble out to the second bottle and the end of the drainage is still sealed with the water so the air does not travel back to the chest (one way valve) (Figure 6.121 - 6.122).

notes...

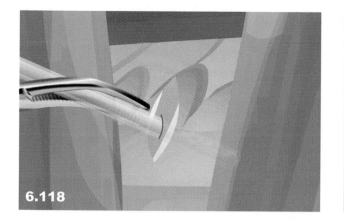

6.118

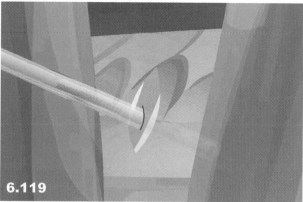

6.119

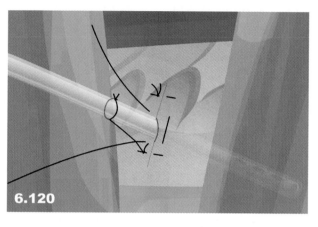

6.120

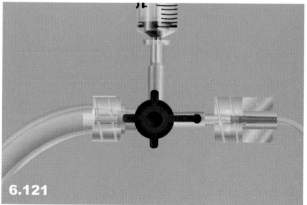

6.121

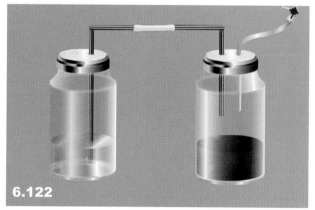

6.122

6:11 Tendon Repair

a) Identify and expose the injury.

b) Irrigate with saline to clear debris.

c) Identify cut end of tendon (Figure 6.123 - 6.126).

d) Handle tendon minimally, do not strip alveolar tissue, minimal debridement.

e) Align and repair using 4-0 or 5-0 Dacron via Kessler modification of Maxon-Allen repair as follows:

• Place stitch into body of tendon longitudinally exiting laterally 1cm from cut edge (Figure 6.127).

• Pass stitch through tendon transversely exiting on the opposite side (Figure 6.128 - 6.129).

• Cut the rough edges of the tendon (Figure 6.130).

(text and illustrations continued on next page)

notes...

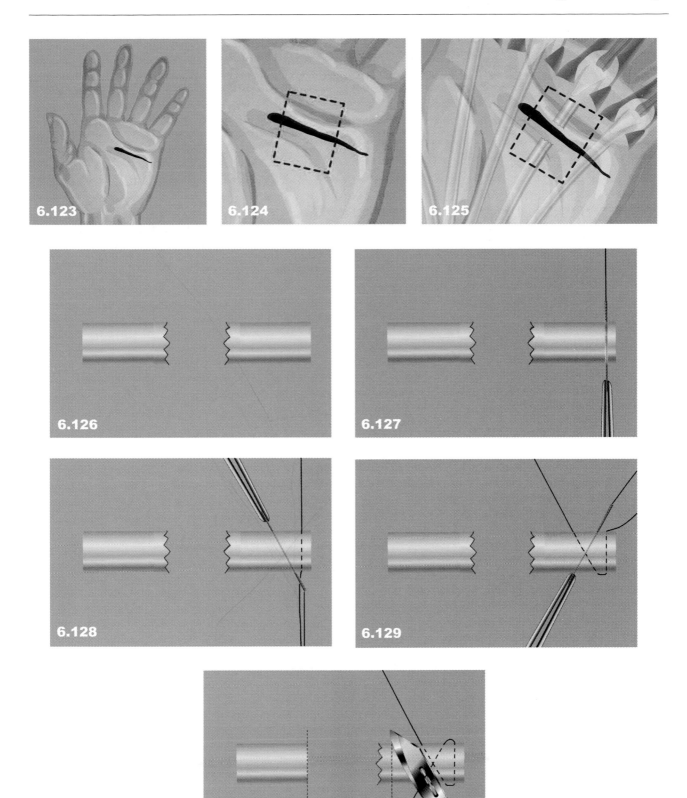

- Pass stitch longitudinally through body of tendon exiting cut surface (Figure 6.131 - 6.132).
- Continue with other end of tendon as for first end (Figure 6.133 - 6.136).
- Knot ends of suture (Figure 6.137).
- Place continuous running sutures of 6-0 nylon in the epitenon to invert edges slightly for a smooth finish.
- Irrigate.
- Close (deep absorbable layer if possible, then superficial non-absorbable interupted).
- Splint limb in position without tension on the repair.

NB: Tendon repair is a very complicated procedure. This section attempts to familiarize one with the sewing technique for tendon repair only. In order to repair tendons properly, more information should be sought elsewhere.

notes...

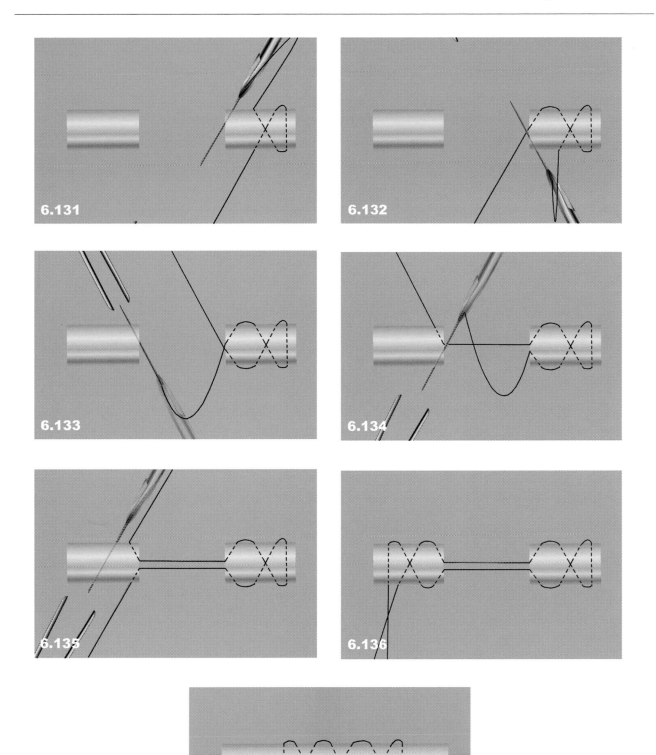

6.131

6.132

6.133

6.134

6.135

6.136

6.137

6:12 Peripheral Nerve Repair (Tibial)

a) Irrigate wound.

b) Identify cut ends of nerve (Figure 6.138).

c) Debride to healthy nerve (Figure 6.139).

d) Align cut ends ensuring no rotation.

e) Release tourniquet to ensure hemostasis.

f) Place a single 8-0 Prolene suture through the perineurium to re-approximate the nerve, leaving the end 3 cm long and held with a bull-dog clamp (Figure 6.140).

g) Place a second suture at 180 degrees to the first (Figure 6.141).

h) Re-approximate the anterior perineurium with interrupted sutures placed 1.5 mm apart (Figure 6.142).

i) Turn the nerve over by passing one bull-dog over and the other under the nerve (Figure 6.143).

j) Repair posterior perineurium as for anterior.

k) Cut excess sutures.

l) Close as for tendon repair.

m) Splint (without tension on repair).

NB: This section describes only the technique for peripheral nerve repair. Detailed information should be sought elsewhere.

notes...

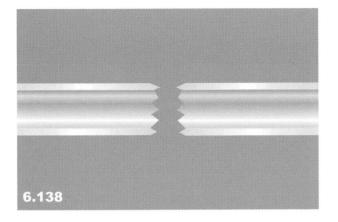

6.138

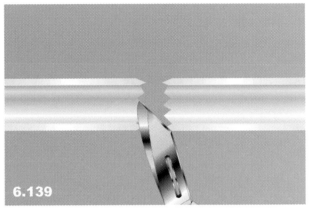

6.139

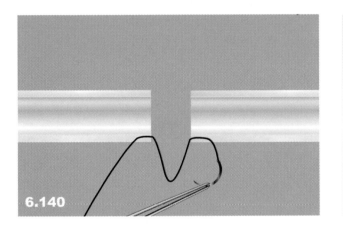

6.140

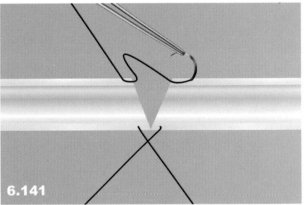

6.141

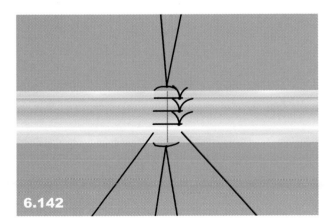

6.142

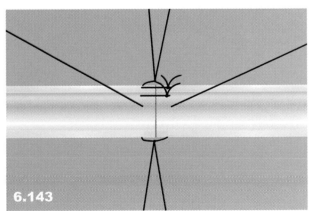

6.143

6:13 Diagnostic Peritoneal Lavage

a) Aseptic techniques

b) Local infiltration anesthesia

c) Location

• umbilical and infra-umbilical area (Figure 6.144 - 6.145), anteroposterior projection

• skin

• superficial fascia

• deep fascia

• linea alba (the aponeuroses of rectus abdominis)

• transverse abdominal muscle

• parietal peritoneum

• peritoneal cavity

d) Incision

• infra-umbilical 2-3 cm (Figure 6.146 - 6.147).

e) Aspirate to detect gross blood or enteric content..

f) Placement of a catheter under direct vision after peritoneum is opened (Figure 6.148-6.150).

g) One litre of normal saline is instilled into the peritoneal cavity and then allowed to drain by gravity.

h) At least 200 ml of lavage fluid should be recovered and sent for analysis.

i) Peritoneum and the wound are closed layer by layer (Figure 6.151).

j) Results are judged by the colour of the fluid and lab analysis.

k) The wound is closed.

notes...

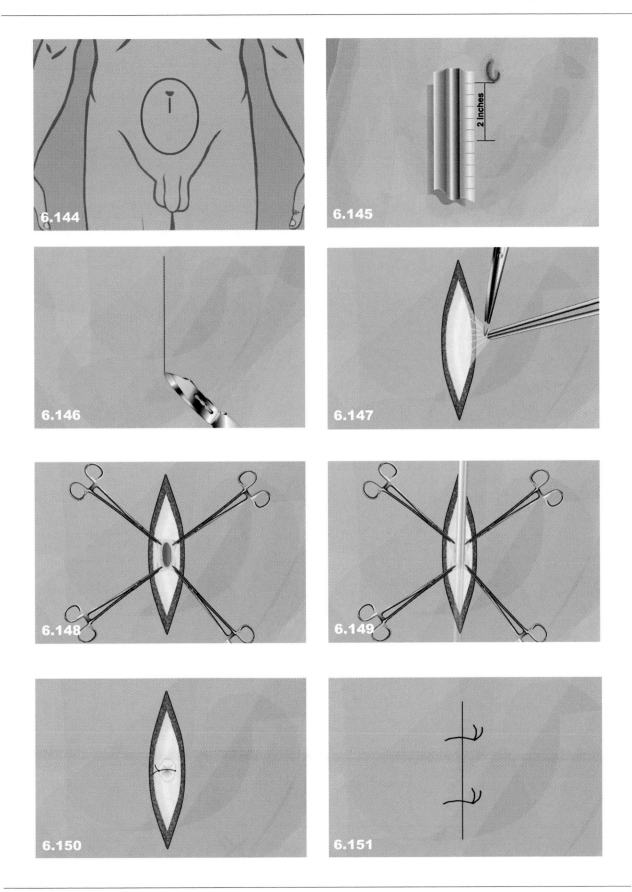

Laparoscopic Surgical Techniques

E.J. Patterson and A.G. Nagy

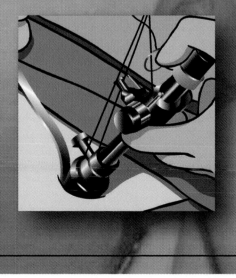

Chapter 7		Contents	Page

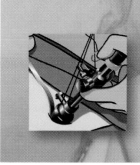

Laparoscopy, or the insertion of an endoscope into the peritoneal cavity, was first described at the beginning of the 20th century. Urologists and gynecologists were pioneers in the development of laparoscopy, where advances in equipment and surgical techniques went hand in hand. The "Laparoscopic Revolution" followed the first descriptions of a completely laparoscopic operation in the late 1980s, the laparoscopic cholecystectomy. Significant patient benefits were realized, in terms of decreased post-operative pain and morbidity, shorter hospital stay, and earlier return to work following laparoscopic cholecystectomy compared with open or conventional cholecystectomy. The current era in surgery is one of "Laparoscopic Evolution", where most surgical procedures are performed partially (laparoscopic-assisted) or completely laparoscopically. However, the scientific evidence of benefits to patient and society, over standard open techniques, is often lacking.

While we await the results of prospective trials to determine the benefits of specific procedures, one thing is certain-laparoscopic surgery is here to stay, and surgeons of the 21st century must possess basic laparoscopic skills.

Videoendoscopic surgery, or the use of fibreoptic scopes, cameras and video monitors to perform surgery in an existing or potential anatomic space, has permeated most of the surgical sub-specialities. Neurosurgeons perform endoscopic surgery within the ventricles. Plastic surgeons perform endoscopic carpal tunnel release in the wrist and also do some facial cosmetic procedures endoscopically. Some surgeons are using the endoscopic approach in the neck for thyroid and parathyroid surgery. Vascular, cardiovascular and thoracic surgeons are also using endoscopic techniques to approach lungs, aortic aneurysms, peripheral vessel and coronary artery bypass grafts.This chapter focuses on basic equipment and techniques used in endoscopic surgery of the peritoneal cavity, ie. laparoscopic surgery.

7:1 Laparoscopic Equipment

Quality, functional equipment is vital to the performance of a successful and efficient laparoscopic operation. The surgeon must be familiar with the equipment and must be able to troubleshoot equipment problems. In fact, the operating room nurses and all surgical personnel should be familiar with the equipment, and the formation of a specialized "Laparoscopic Team" is likely the most efficient solution.

7:1:1 Laparoscopes

The standard laparoscope in general surgery is 10 mm in diameter, whereas gynecologists often use slightly smaller 7 mm scopes. The angle of the lens may be 0 degree (looking end-on) or angled at 30 degrees or greater. Most surgeons find the 30 degree scope provides an excellent view for basic laparoscopic procedures. Recently, smaller "mini-laparoscopes" of 1.5 to 3.5 mm in diameter have been introduced, which may be of either fibre optic or rod-lens construction.

7:1:2 Video

Today, the term 'laparoscopy' implies 'videolaparoscopy', or the attachment of a video camera to the lighted telescope into the abdomen. Initially, laparoscopy was performed with the surgeon looking directly into the eyepiece of the scope, held inside the patient's abdomen. Now virtually all laparoscopy is videolaparoscopy where the image is displayed on a video monitor. Hence there is surgical hand-eye separation which contributes to the technical difficulty of laparoscopic surgery.

It is often advantageous to have two monitors, one on each side of the operating table. The specific position of video monitors depends on the operation. In general the monitors are located on the pathology side, and the surgeon stands across the table, facing the video. The video cassette recorder, video monitor, light source and gas insufflator are usually housed in a single tower (Figure 7.1).

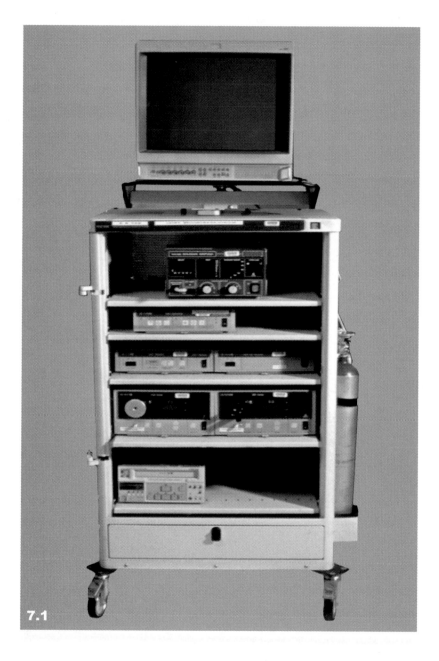

7.1

7:1:3 Light Source

Early laparoscopes used an incandescent light bulb at the tip of the scope. The development of fiber optics has led to the movement of the light source and its controls to a separate and distant unit connected to the endoscope with a light cord (Figure 7.2a).

7:1:4 Gas Insufflator

Gas insufflation of the peritoneal cavity converts the potential space into an actual one, several litres in size. Gas flow is continuous with an adjustable rate (up to 6 - 10 L/min) and maximum pressure control (maximum 12-15 mmHg recommended).
Carbon dioxide is the most commonly used insufflation gas since it is rapidly absorbed into the circulation, thus minimizing the potential for gas embolism. Nitrous oxide has been used under local anesthesia since it is purported to be less irritating to the peritoneum. The disadvantage of nitrous oxide is that it supports combustion, preventing the use of cautery, and thus limiting its usefulness as an insufflation gas.

Special laparoscopic retractors of the anterior abdominal wall ("abdominal wall lifters") permit creation of a potential space without continuous gas insufflation, theoretically decreasing the potential for gas embolism. Abdominal wall lifters have been advocated when large blood vessels such as

hepatic veins are being transected, but there is no good evidence to support their use.

7:1:5 Laparoscopic Instruments

Many laparoscopic instruments are modifications of standard surgical instruments. The tips are finer and are mounted on long (30 cm) shafts to pass through the abdominal wall to the operative site. Other laparoscopic instruments are unique in that they do not have counterparts in open surgery (e.g. L-hook and spatula cautery instruments). Instruments which rely on sharp surfaces may be either reusable or disposable. Disposable instruments have the advantage of staying sharper but the disadvantage of higher cost.

a) Veress Needle. A needle for obtaining closed access to the peritoneal cavity in order to create a pneumoperitoneum. It has a spring-loaded obturator which retracts to expose the sharp tip while there is resistance passing through the abdominal wall, and advances over the needle tip upon entering the peritoneal cavity (Figure 7.2b).

b) Hasson Cannula. A device for establishing open access to the peritoneal cavity. This consists of a 10 cm blunt trocar and 11 mm cannula which can be fastened to the abdominal wall to prevent gas leakage or cannula slippage (Figure 7.2c).

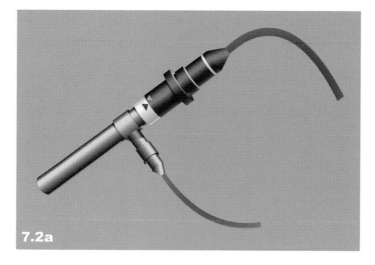

7.2a

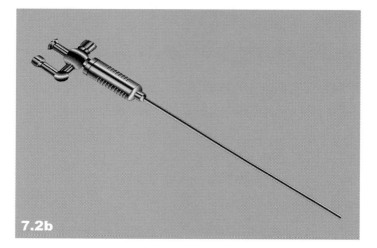

7.2b

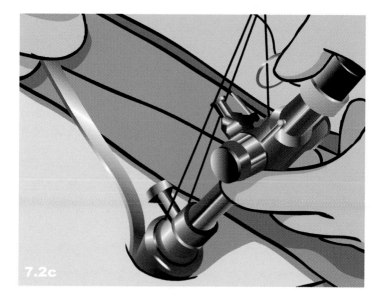

7.2c

c) Trocars and Cannulas. Fundamental tools of laparoscopic surgery which provide and maintain access to the peritoneal cavity for the insertion of operating instruments. A cannula is a hollow tube of various diameters (3-20 mm, commonly 5 or 11 mm). This is placed through the abdominal wall with a sharp inner trocar which is then removed. Trocars are either metal (reusable) , plastic (disposable), or a hybrid of the two with a reusable cannula and a plastic trocar (Figure 7.3).

d) Scissors. Scissors are used for sharp or blunt dissection, with or without electrocautery. Varieties include straight, curved and hook scissors. Hook scissors are designed so that the tips come together prior to the cutting surface so that a tubular structure can be grasped and then held away from surrounding tissue for safe cutting (Figure 7.4).

e) Graspers. Numerous different types of graspers are available for grasping tissue or specimens such as gallstones. These can be traumatic or atraumatic (with or without teeth), and with or without a ratcheted handle that keeps the jaws closed without manual pressure (Figure 7.5). The tripod grasper is useful for grasping a thick-walled gallbladder (Figure 7.6).

f) Dissectors. Multiple different types with similar designs to open instruments. Fine straight dissector, Maryland and Mixter are shown here (Figure 7.7).

g) Cautery Tips. A variety of shapes of cautery tips are available for monopolar electrocautery dissection. The most common varieties are the L-hook and spatula (Figure 7.8).

h) Needle Drivers. Laparoscopic needle drivers are similar to standard needle drivers (Figure 7.9). As opposed to most instruments which have pistol-grip handles, needle drivers usually have co-axial handles to facilitate "palming" the instrument. (Figure 7.10).

notes...

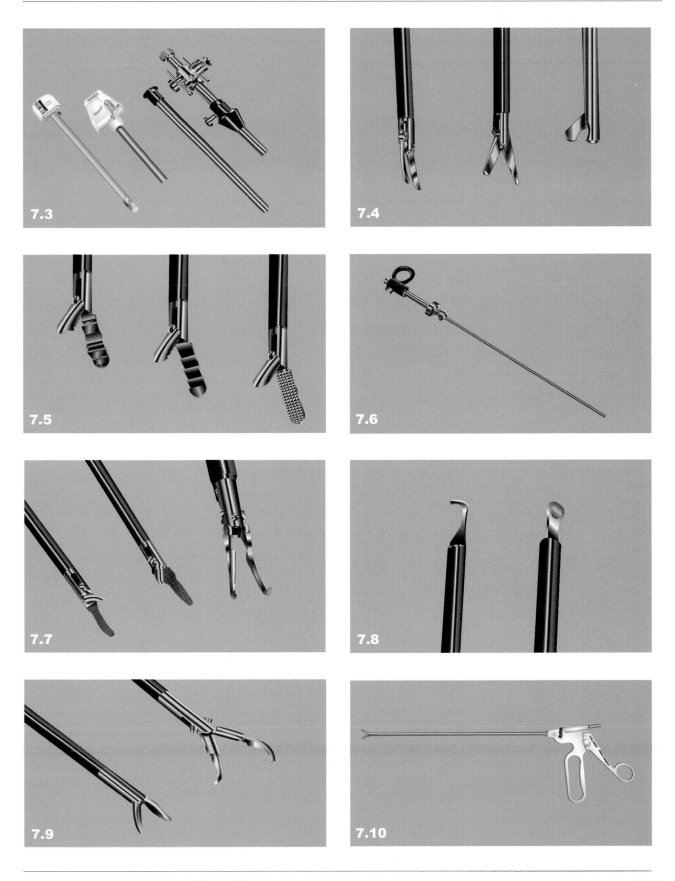

i) Endoloop. Pre-tied ligature used for controlling blind-ended structures such as the appendix. An endoloop may also be placed over the end of a structure previously clipped and cut where the clip may be inadequate alone (i.e. large cystic duct) (Figure 7.11).

j) Suction and irrigation device. Important instrument for keeping the operative field clean and dry (blood is magnified on the screen, and the dark colour not only absorbs the light but directly obscures anatomy) (Figure 7.12).

k) Endoscopic stapler. Similar uses as in open surgery, but requires a 12 mm cannula (Figure 7.13). This fires two double rows of staples and cuts between them.

7:1:6 Operating Table Set-Up

Sterile drape the patient widely to maximize flexibility of port site positions. Port sites represent a finite number of views of the operative field. Choose them wisely but do not feel restricted in adding extra ports as needed. However, extra ports actually add little extra morbidity. Several animal and clinical studies have concluded that the physiologic stress of one long incision appears to be greater than that of several short incisions of the same total incision length.

Plan position of patient, surgeon, assistant, scrub nurse, and videolaparoscopic equipment, and organize the "cables" accordingly. A suction and irrigation device should be immediately available for any laparoscopic case i.e. setup, and turned on.

notes...

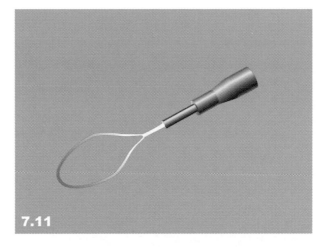

7.11

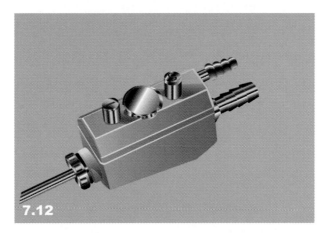

7.12

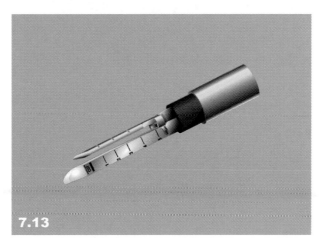

7.13

7:2 Handling Laparoscopic Instruments

Most laparoscopic instruments have finger ring or pistol grips, and are generally handled similar to standard surgical instruments.

General Principles:

a) Two-Handed Technique. It is at least as important in laparoscopic as in open surgery for the surgeon to use both hands simultaneously. The principle of traction and counter-traction requires constant repositioning of the non-dominant hand.

b) Camera Operator. This critical member of the laparoscopic team functions as the surgeons' eyes. A good camera person is essential for consistent visualization throughout the procedure. The structure or organ which the surgeon is manipulating should be kept in the centre of the screen. If the surgeon is satisfied with the view, the camera should be kept still. Any camera movements should be small, and should be made slowly and smoothly, in order to avoid inducing motion sickness in those watching the monitor. The black cord coming off the end of the camera sets the "horizon" of the view, and therefore should always be kept down, toward the ground so that the surgeon remains oriented to the anatomy (Figure 7.14).

The gray light cord entering the side of the angled laparoscope adjusts the direction of the angle. The camera angle is always looking away from the cord.

c) Instrument Changes. These are time consuming and should be minimized. Novice laparoscopists should have their instruments escorted by the camera from the port to the target structure to be operated upon. Experienced laparoscopists can triangulate the ports in order to safely move the instrument in and out of the abdomen without moving the camera, except perhaps to zoom out slightly to view the inserted instrument. An important job of the assistant is to hold the cannula steady while the surgeon inserts the instrument.

notes...

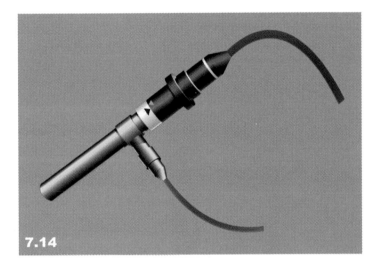

7.14

7:3 Basic Laparoscopic Techniques

The key to success and consistency in performing any laparoscopic procedure, including these basic techniques, is to establish a routine.

7:3:1 Pneumoperitoneum

The pneumoperitoneum is the laparoscopists' workspace. Without the distension of this potential space, laparoscopic surgery is not possible. There are two basic techniques of establishing access to the peritoneal cavity and creating a pneumoperitoneum.

Proponents of the Veress technique argue that it is quick and easy. Surgeons in favour of the Hasson technique counter that it is safer since everything is done under direct vision, and that the rapid insufflation makes up for the extra time required to insert a Hasson cannula compared with a Veress needle. Some surgeons selectively use either technique, using the Veress needle in uncomplicated cases and the open technique when adhesions from previous surgery are anticipated.

a) Veress Needle (Closed Technique)

• Infiltrate local anesthetic below the umbilicus (Figure 7.15).

• Make a skin incision the size of the port to be inserted (Figure 7.16).
• Grasp the fascia with a hemostat or towel-clip and retract upwards (Figure 7.17).
• Insert the Veress needle through all layers of the abdominal wall; there should be two distinct "pops" (Figure 7.18).
• Tests for intraperitoneal location:

  -Aspirate. First aspirate (for blood or bowel content, which would identify a serious trocar-entry complication), then flush with 5 cc saline and aspirate again (Figure 7.19)

  -Hanging Drop. Place a drop of saline in the hub of the Veress, then lift the abdominal wall. If the Veress is in place the negative intra-abdominal pressure should pull the drop inwards, and disappear inside the needle.

• Insufflate with CO_2, first on low flow then increase when sure that the flow is in the intraperitoneum. This location can be confirmed by percussing over the liver (normal dullness is lost due to the pneumoperitoneum) (Figure 7.20)
• Insert the first sharp trocar, with the side port open so that the "hiss" of escaping air can be heard when the pneumoperitoneum is penetrated (forward pressure on the port is immediately released, and the side port is closed to prevent loss of the pneumoperitoneum) (Figure 7.21).

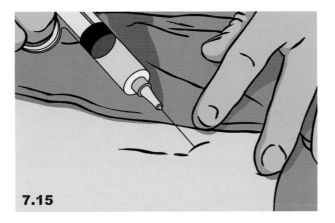

7.15

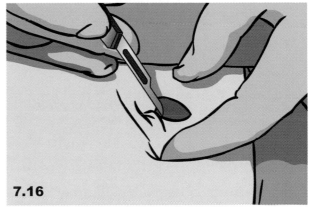

7.16

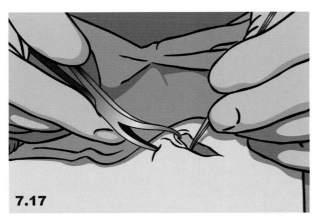

7.17

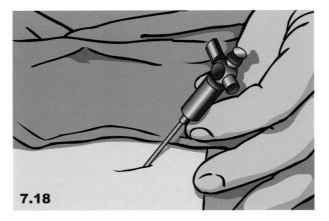

7.18

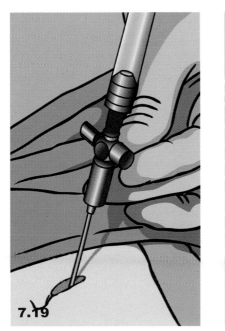

7.19

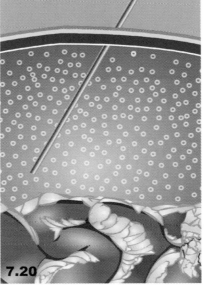

7.20

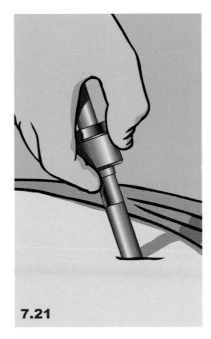

7.21

b) Hasson Cannula (Open Technique)

• Infiltrate local anesthetic below the umbilicus.

• Make a skin incision 12-15 mm long for a 10 mm Hasson. The thicker the abdominal wall, the longer the incision will be.

• Grasp the fascia with a hemostat or towel-clip and retract upwards (Figure 7.22).

• Make a 10 mm incision in all layers of fascia (the linea alba) (Figure 7.23).

• Open the peritoneum (either sharply between two hemostats, or bluntly with the gloved finger) (Figure 7.24).

• Place "stay sutures" in the fascia which will be used to achieve a tight seal between the abdominal wall and the cannula to prevent gas escape. Place the sutures so that they can be used to close the fascial defect after the procedure (to prevent a trocar site herniation) (Figure 7.25).

• Insert the Hasson using an S-retractor to visualize the path into the peritoneal cavity (think of this as "intubating" the peritoneal cavity) (Figure 7.26).

• Fasten the Hasson in place with the stay sutures and insufflate with CO_2. High flow can be used immediately as the intraperitoneal location is visualized directly (Figure 7.27).

notes...

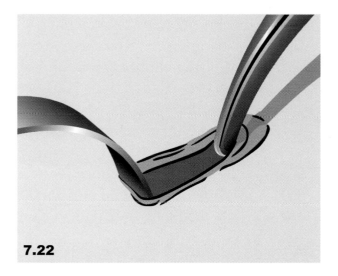

7.22

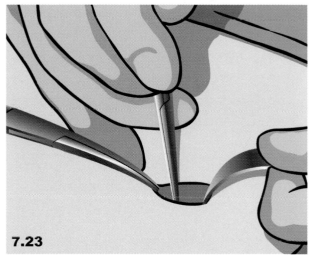

7.23

7.24

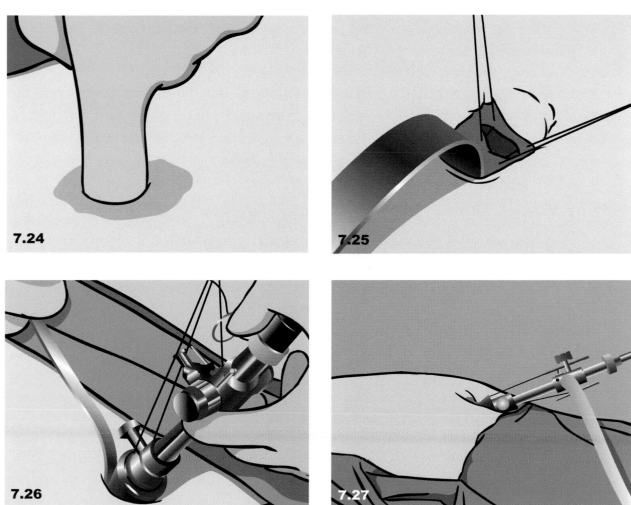

7.25

7.26

7.27

7:3:2 Basic Laparoscopic Skills

As with traditional surgery, the basic principles of laparoscopic surgery are traction and counter-traction, and meticulous sharp and blunt dissection. The difference between the two is the very fine hand movements required for laparoscopic dissection, as instruments are restricted in movement around a fulcrum at the abdominal wall.

Very basic surgical techniques such as knot-tying therefore become much more difficult. In fact, many surgeons would realistically consider laparoscopic intracorporeal knot-tying an advanced laparoscopic technique. It is definitely a prerequisite skill for advanced laparoscopic surgery (i.e. in general surgery, anything beyond cholecystectomy, appendectomy, or inguinal hernia repair).

Due to the difficulty of laparoscopic suturing, novel techniques have developed for laparoscopic hemostasis (e.g. "endoloops") and other traditional techniques have adapted to laparoscopic surgery. Only those skills which are important or unique in laparoscopic surgery will be described in this section. These skills can be practiced in dry (inanimate) and wet (animate) labs.

a) Transfer. Hand-to-hand transfer of a needle from right hand to left hand and vice versa. Hand-over-hand movements required to "run the bowel" can be simulated by a piece of string in a laparoscopic practice box.

b) Clipping a Vessel. The basic principle of having the tips of the instrument in view at all times is paramount . The surgeon must see the tips of the clip during application (Figures 7.28 - 7.30).

c) Dissection. Sharp or blunt dissection with or without cautery, as in open surgery (Figures 7.31 & 7.32). In addition, tissues are picked up, lifted away from surrounding structures, coagulated, and then stripped away to expose the underlying structure (Figures 7.33 & 7.34). Small vessels can also be grasped, cauterized, and then sharply divided with scissors (Figures 7.35 - 7.37).

d) Applying an Endoloop
• "Backload" the endoloop into the reducer.
• Insert the endoloop into the abdomen.
• Place the loop over the target structure to be ligated.
• Grasp the target with a ratcheted instrument in the other hand, and provide counter-traction (the assistant holds this instrument so that the surgeon can use two hands on the endoloop).
• Snap off the end of the endoloop, place the tip of the holder on the desired position of the ligature and smoothly pull the suture to snug down the loop.
• Cut the suture and remove the endoloop holder. Small vessels can also be grasped, cauterized, and then sharply divided with scissors.

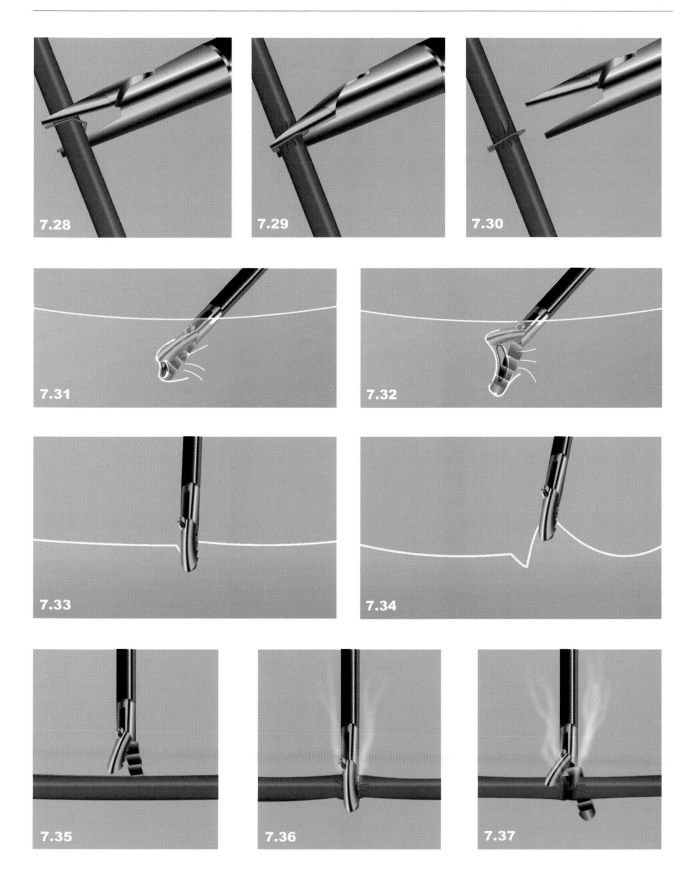

7.28

7.29

7.30

7.31

7.32

7.33

7.34

7.35

7.36

7.37

7:3:3 Laparoscopic Suturing

Curved needles are commonly used for suturing in open surgery. Some surgeons prefer short, straight needles or ski-tip needles when they are learning laparoscopic suturing techniques.

a) Intracorporeal Knots. Intracorporeal knots are laparoscopic instrument ties formed completely within the peritoneal cavity. This is essentially an instrument tie, as in open surgery, but it is much more difficult to do laparoscopically. Due to the technical difficulty of this basic laparoscopic skill, many surgeons have abandoned it in favour of the easier extracorporeal suturing. As with any skill, intracorporeal knot-tying can be mastered with practice.

• Insert the suture (trimmed to a length of about four to six inches) into the abdomen and grasp it in the needle holder (positioned at a right angle to the jaw of the needle holder).
• Pass the needle through the tissue (Figure 7.38).
• Pick up the needle with the second instrument (second needle holder or a swan-neck grasper) and turn over 180 degrees so that the point faces the direction from which the needle came (to reduce the risk of inadvertent injury with the needle while pulling the suture through (Figure 7.39).

• Pull the suture though the tissue in the direction of the needle path (to minimize tissue trauma - as in open surgery) leaving a "tail" of one or two inches of suture protruding from the tissue (Figure 7.40).
• Grasp the suture just beyond the swage (Figure 7.41) and a C-shaped curve is formed with the suture. The needle end of the suture is then wrapped around the second instrument twice (Figure 7.42), the tail is then grasped (Figure 7.43), and the knot is laid down flatly, as with an open instrument tie (Figure 7.44).
• Tighten the first knot and then hand the suture to the opposite instrument and tie a single knot in the opposite direction, resulting in a square knot. At least three knots are usually placed (Figures 7.45 - 7.48).
• Cut the suture and remove excess.

notes...

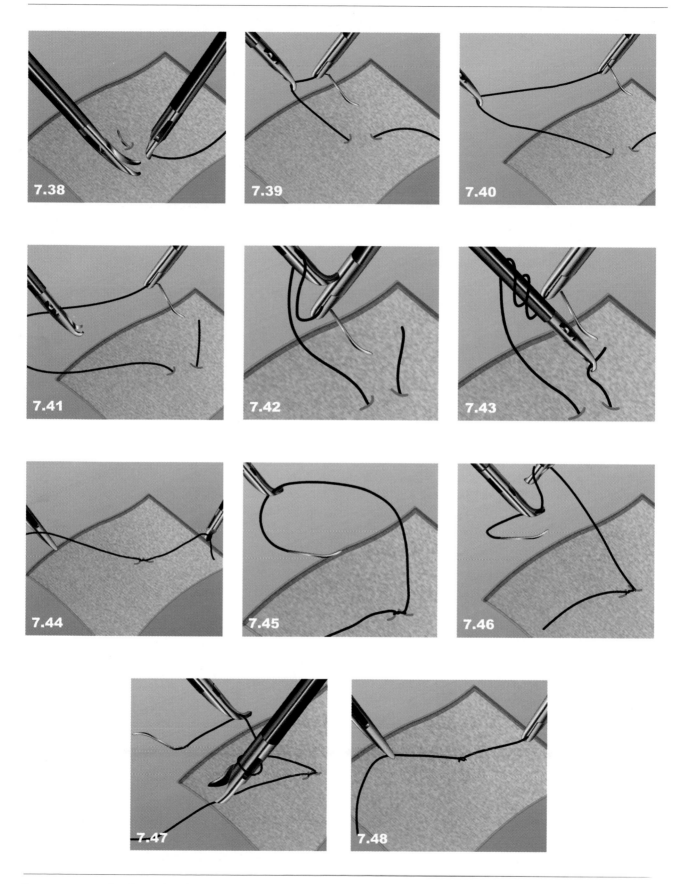

b) Extracorporeal Knots. As the name implies, extracorporeal knot-tying involves the tying of knots outside of the body: The suture and needle are passed into the abdomen, placed through the tissue, pulled out of the abdomen, tied, and pushed back into the abdomen and snugged down.

There are two basic types of extracorporeal knots: extracorporeal slip knots and extracorporeal surgeon's knots (Figures 7.49 - 7.57).

• Insert the suture into the abdomen and grasp it in the needle holder (positioned at a right angle to the jaw of the needle holder).
• Pass the needle through the tissue.
• Grasp the suture behind the swage and pull the needle and the suture back into the trocar sheath through which it was inserted.
• Tie a single knot, while the assistant holds a finger over the trocar sheath opening in order to prevent the escape of gas.
• Use a knot-pusher to push the knot down through the cannula, and onto the tissue (the knot-pusher should be considered an extension of the surgeon's finger, used to push knots down in open surgery). If the surgeon does not wish to use a slip knot, then a surgeon's knot is pushed down, and two or three additional knots are tied and pushed down in succession.
• Cut the suture and remove excess.

notes...

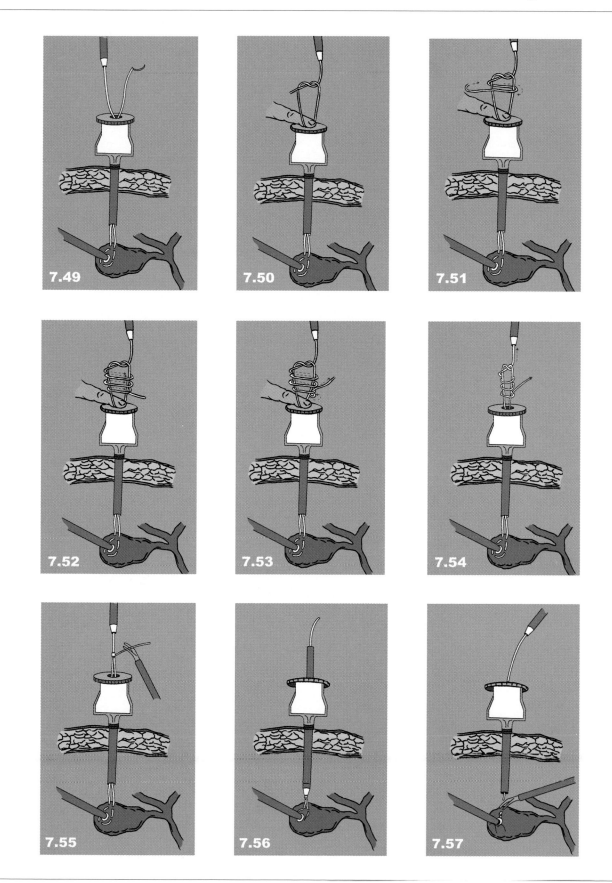

References

1. Agur AMR: Grant's Atlas of Anatomy. Williams and Wilkins 9th ed, Philadelphia. pp650.

2. Anderson RM, Romth F: Techniques in Use of Surgical Tools. Appleton and Lange, Norwalk, Connecticut: 1990:pp211.

3. Annunziata CC, Drake DB, Woods JA, Gear AJ, Rodeheaver GT, Edlich RF. J Emerg Med. 1997 May-Jun:15(3);351-6.

4. Annunziata CC, Drake DB, Woods JA, Gear AJ, Rodeheaver GT, Edlich RF. Technical considerations in knot construction Part I – continuous percutaneous and dermal suture closure. J Emerg Med. 1997 May-Jun:15(3);351-6.

5. Aston SJ: The choice of suture material for skin closure, J Dermatol Surg 1976:2(1);57-61.

6. Athanasiou KA, Niederauer GG, Agrawal CM. Sterilization, toxicity, biocompatibility and clinical applications of polylactic acid/polycolic acid copolymers. Biomaterials. Jan 1996:17(2);93-102.

7. Atkinson LJ, Fortunato N: Barry and Kohn's Operating Room Techniques. Mosby 8th ed, 1999:pp988;163-295.

8. Boltri M. Atraumatic closure of skin wounds with fasterzip. Immediate and long term esthetic results. Minerva Chir. 1997 Nov:52(11);1405-9.

9. Brokaw A, Ellwood L. Planning for pediatric laceration repairs. Nurse Prac. 1996 Mar:21(3);42,45,49.

10. Casha JN, Hadden WA. Suture reaction following skin closure with subcuticular polydioxanone in total knee arthroplasty. J Arthroplasty. 1996 Oct:11(7);859-61.

11. Charbit Y, Hitzig C, Bolla M, Bitton C. Bertrand MF. Comparative study of physical properties of three suture materials: silk, e-PTFE (Gore-Tex) and PLA/PGA (Vicryl). Biomed Instrum Technol. 1999 Jan-Feb:33(1);71-5.

12. Cnota MA, Aliabadi-Wahle S, Choe EU, Jacob JT, Flint LM, Ferrara JJ. Development of a novel synthetic material to close abdominal wall defects. Am Surg. 1998 May:64(5);415-8.

13. Crikelair GF. Skin suture marks. Am J Surg 1958;96:631-9.

14. Debus ES, Geiger D, Sailer M, Ederer J, Thiede A. Physical, biological and handling characteristics of surgical suture material: a comparison of four different multifilament absorbable sutures. Eur Surg Res. 1997:29(1);52-61.

15. Debus ES, Geiger D, Sailer M, Ederer J, Thiede A. Physical, biological and handling characteristics of surgical suture material: a comparison of four different multifilament absorbable sutures. Eur Surg Res. 1997:29(1);52-61.

16. Dripps RD, Eckenhoff JE, Vandam LD: Introduction to Anesthesia – the principles of safe practice. W.B. Saunders Co, 1992:pp557;242-288.

17. Eden CG, Coptcoat MJ. Assessment of alternative tissue approximation techniques for laparoscopy. Br J Urol. 1996 Aug:78(2);234-42.

18. Eriesson BF: Basic Techniques in Vascular Surgery. Davis and Geck, USA. 1988:pp56.

19. Evans RB. An update on wound management. Hand Clin. 1991 Aug: Vol.7#3:409-432.

20. Forrester JC, Zederfeldt BH, Hayes TL et al. Tape-closed and sutured wounds; a comparison by tensiometry and scanning electron microscope. Br J Surg 1970: 57(10);729-37.

21. Gawenda M, Prokop A. Treatment strategies in bite injuries. Langenbecks Arch Chir - supplement. Kongressband. 1997:114-521-7.

22. Ger R. The use of external tissue expansion in the management of wounds and ulcers. Ann Plast Surg. 1997 Apr:38(4);352-7.

23. Hau T, Forster E. Treatment of Surgical Wounds: facts and fiction. Zentralbl Chir. 1996:121 suppl:39-40.

24. Hightower D, March J, Ausband S, Brown LH. Comparison of staples vs suturing for securing central venous catheters. Acad Emerg Med. Dec 1996:3(12);1103-5.

25. Hinrichsen N, Birk-Sorensen L, Gottrup F, Hjortdal V. Wound contraction in an experimental porcine model. Scand J Plast Reconstr Hand Surg. 1998 Sep: 32(3);243-8.

26. Hollander JE, Singer AJ, Valentine S. Comparison of wound care practices in pediatric and adult lacerations repaired in the emergency department. Pediatr Emerg Care. 1998 Feb:14(1);15-8.

27. Howell JM, Chisholm CD. Wound care. Emerg Med Clin North Am. 1997 May:15(2);417-25.

28. Israelsson LA, Jonsson T, Knutsson A. Suture technique and wound healing in midline laparotomy incisions. Eur J Sur. 1996 Aug:162(8);605-9

29. Israelsson LA, Jonsson T. Overweight and healing of midline incisions: the importance of suture techniques. Eur J Surg. 1997 Mar:163(3);175-80.

30. Kaplan JA: Cardiac Anesthesia. Grune and Stratton – a subsidiary of Harcourt Brace Joranovith Publishers. New York: 1995: pp529;p473-501.

31. Kratz G. Modeling of wound healing processes in human skin using tissue culture. Microsc Res Tech. 1998 Sep: 42(5);345-50.

32. Le TB, Mizel MS, Temple HT. Reducing post-surgical pain and tissue reaction from suture-induced skin tenting. Foot Ankle Int. Jun 1998:19(6);420

33. Leppaniemi AK, Wherry DC, Soltero RG, Pikoulis E, Hufnagel HV et al. A quick and simple method to close vascular, biliary and urinary tract incisions using the new Vascular Closure Staples: a preliminary report. Surg Endosc. 1996 Jul: 10(7);771-4.

34. Mackrodt C, Gordon B, Fern E, Ayers S, Truesdale A, Grant A. The Ipswich Childbirth Study: A randomised comparison of polyglactin 910 with chromic catgut for postpartum perineal repair. Br J Obstet Gynaecol. 1998 Apr: 105(4);441-5.

35. Meeker MH, Rothroek JC: Alexander's Care of the Patient in Surgery. Mosby 11th ed, 1999:pp1380;3-273.

36. Memisoglu E, Oner F, Ayhan A, Basaran I, Hincal AA. In vivo evaluation for rhGM-CSF wound-healing efficacy in topical vehicles. Pharma Develop Tech. 1997 May:2(2);171-80.

37. Moy RL, Waldman B, Hein DWA: Review of sutures and suturing techniques. J Dematol Surg Oncol 1992;18(9):785-95.

38. Nagy A. Surgical Laparoscopy Update 2nd ed. Zucker KA editor. 1993: Quality Medical Publishing.

39. Nealon TF: Fundamental skills in Surgery 2nd ed. WB Saunders Co. p53-4;1971.
40. Outlaw KK, Vela AR, O'Leary JP. Breaking strength and diameter of absorbable sutures after in vivo exposure in the rat. Am Surg. 1998 Apr:64(4);348-54.

41. Partridge C. Influential factors in surgical wound healing. J Wound Care. 1998 Jul:7(7);350-3.

42. Quilici PJ: New Developments in Laparoscopy. USSC, Canada: 1992:pp152.

43. Schnall SB, Thommen VD, Allari T, Holtom PD. Delayed primary wound closure in upper extremity soft tissue infections. Clin Orthop 1997 Feb:(335);286-91.

44. Selvadurai D, Wildin C, Treharne G. Choksy SA, Heywood MM et al. Randomised trial of subcuticular suture versus metal clips for wound closure after thyroid and parathyroid surgery. Comment in Ann R Coll Surg Engl. 1997 Nov:79(6);469

45. Shatalov AD. Nonabsorbable suture material as a source of biliary calculi formation. Klin Khir. 1998: (3)16-7

46. Sinclair RD, Ryan TJ, Proteolytic enzymes in wound healing. The role of enzymatic debridement. Australas J Dermatol. 1994:35;41.

47. Skripnikov NS, Kostenko VA, Pronina EN, Romantsev A. Morphological and metabolic changes in tissues during surgical suture implantation. Klin Khir. 1997:(11-12);78-81.

48. Soroff HS, Harman AR, Pak E, Sasvary DH, Pollak SB. Improved sternal closure using steel bands: early experience with three-year follow-up. Ann Thorac Surg. 1996 Apr:61(4);1172-6.

49. Spotnitz WD, Falstrom JK, Rodeheaver GT. The role of sutures and fibrin sealant in wound healing. Surg Clin North Am. Jun 1997:77(3);651-69.

50. Synder CC: On the history of the suture. Plas Recon Surg 1976:58(4):401-6.

51. Usgaocar RP. Lessening the pain of suture removal. Comments. Plast Reconstr Surg. 1998 Jul:102(1);268.

52. Way LW: Current Surgical Diagnosis and Treatment. Appletion and Lange, Norwalk, Connecticut: 1994:pp1425;27,198,887, 203-5.

53. Zatit SC, Mazzer N, Barbieri CH. Mechanical Strengths of tendon sutures - an in vitro comparative study of six techniques. J Hand Surg – British Volume. 1998 May:23(2);228-33.

54. Zikria B. Knot Tying Manual. Ethicon Inc. Somerville, NJ 1998:40.

55. Zollinger and Zollinger: Atlas of Surgical Operation. McGraw-Hill Inc. 7th ed. New York, 1999:pp484;388.

Index

Basic Surgical Techniques **Order Form**

I would like to order the book *Basic Surgical Techniques* by A.K. Qayumi.

Name _____

Address _____

City, State/Province _____

Country/Zip/Postal Code _____

I enclose a ☐ personal cheque   ☐ bank draft

Please charge to: ☐ Amex   ☐ Visa   ☐ MasterCard   (issuing bank # _____)

Account # _____ Exp. _____ Signature _____

The price for *Basic Surgical Techniques* is $150.00 U.S.
Please include $5.00 shipping/handling within North America, $10.00 outside North America.
Mail to: *Basic Surgical Techniques,* 1170-West 7th Ave., Vancouver, BC, Canada, V6H 1B4
You can also fax your order to us at (604) 875-5832.
For faster service, telephone (604) 730-8255.

Basic Surgical Techniques **Order Form**

I would like to order the book *Basic Surgical Techniques* by A.K. Qayumi.

Name _____

Address _____

City, State/Province _____

Country/Zip/Postal Code _____

I enclose a ☐ personal cheque   ☐ bank draft

Please charge to: ☐ Amex   ☐ Visa   ☐ MasterCard   (issuing bank # _____)

Account # _____ Exp. _____ Signature _____

The price for *Basic Surgical Techniques* is $150.00 U.S.
Please include $5.00 shipping/handling within North America, $10.00 outside North America.
Mail to: *Basic Surgical Techniques,* 1170-West 7th Ave., Vancouver, BC, Canada, V6H 1B4
You can also fax your order to us at (604) 875-5832.
For faster service, telephone (604) 730-8255.

Basic Surgical Techniques **Order Form**

I would like to order the book *Basic Surgical Techniques* by A.K. Qayumi.

Name _____

Address _____

City, State/Province _____

Country/Zip/Postal Code _____

I enclose a ☐ personal cheque   ☐ bank draft

Please charge to: ☐ Amex   ☐ Visa   ☐ MasterCard   (issuing bank # _____)

Account # _____ Exp. _____ Signature _____

The price for *Basic Surgical Techniques* is $150.00 U.S.
Please include $5.00 shipping/handling within North America, $10.00 outside North America.
Mail to: *Basic Surgical Techniques,* 1170-West 7th Ave., Vancouver, BC, Canada, V6H 1B4
You can also fax your order to us at (604) 875-5832.
For faster service, telephone (604) 730-8255.

This book is considered to be one of the best sources of information on basic surgical techniques by peers, undergraduate students and surgical residents. It is designed to discuss the practical aspects of basic surgical skills required for MDs, surgical assistants or nurses. This book consists of seven chapters, more than 500 colour illustrations and is accompanied by an interactive CD-ROM that contains more than 100 colour animations. To have a closer look at the book, visit our website at www.surgical-techniques.com. For faster delivery, please call 604-730-8255.

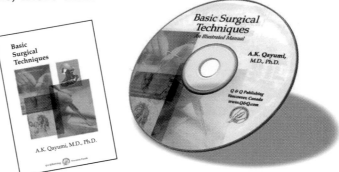

This book is considered to be one of the best sources of information on basic surgical techniques by peers, undergraduate students and surgical residents. It is designed to discuss the practical aspects of basic surgical skills required for MDs, surgical assistants or nurses. This book consists of seven chapters, more than 500 colour illustrations and is accompanied by an interactive CD-ROM that contains more than 100 colour animations. To have a closer look at the book, visit our website at www.surgical-techniques.com. For faster delivery, please call 604-730-8255.

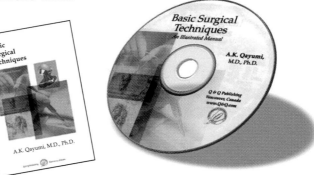

This book is considered to be one of the best sources of information on basic surgical techniques by peers, undergraduate students and surgical residents. It is designed to discuss the practical aspects of basic surgical skills required for MDs, surgical assistants or nurses. This book consists of seven chapters, more than 500 colour illustrations and is accompanied by an interactive CD-ROM that contains more than 100 colour animations. To have a closer look at the book, visit our website at www.surgical-techniques.com. For faster delivery, please call 604-730-8255.

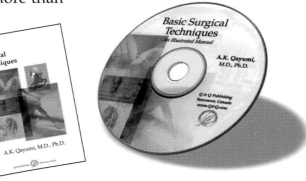